BEING AND BELONGING

WILEY SERIES IN PSYCHOTHERAPY AND COUNSELLING

SERIES EDITORS
Franz Epting, *Dept of Psychology, University of Florida, USA*
Bonnie Strickland, *Dept of Psychology, University of Massachusetts, USA*
John Allen, *Dept of Community Studies, University of Brighton, UK*

Self, Symptoms and Psychotherapy
Edited by Neil Cheshire and Helmut Thomae

Beyond Sexual Abuse: Therapy with Women who were Childhood Victims
Derek Jehu

Cognitive-Analytic Therapy: Active Participation in Change: A New Integration in Brief Psychotherapy
Anthony Ryle

The Power of Countertransference: Innovations in Analytic Technique
Karen J. Maroda

Strategic Family Play Therapy
Shlomo Ariel

The Evolving Professional Self: Stages and Themes in Therapist and Counselor Development
Thomas M. Skovholt and Michael Helge Rønnestad

Feminist Perspectives in Therapy: An Empowerment Model for Women
Judith Worell and Pam Remer

Counselling and Therapy with Refugees: Psychological Problems of Victims of War, Torture and Repression
Guus van der Veer

Psychoanalytic Counseling
Michael J. Patton and Naomi M. Meara

Life Stories: Personal Construct Therapy with the Elderly
Linda L. Viney

The Therapeutic Relationship in Behavioural Psychotherapy
Cas Schaap, Ian Bennun, Ludwig Schindler and Kees Hoogduin

Being and Belonging: Group, Intergroup and Gestalt
Gaie Houston

Further titles in preparation

BEING AND BELONGING
Group, Intergroup and Gestalt

Gaie Houston

JOHN WILEY & SONS
Chichester · New York · Brisbane · Toronto · Singapore

Copyright © 1993 Gaie Houston

Published 1993 by John Wiley & Sons Ltd,
Baffins Lane, Chichester
West Sussex PO19 1UD, England

All rights reserved.

No part of this book may be reproduced by any means,
or transmitted, or translated into a machine language
without the written permission of the publisher.

Other Wiley Editorial Offices

John Wiley & Sons, Inc., 605 Third Avenue,
New York, NY 10158-0012, USA

Jacaranda Wiley Ltd, G.P.O. Box 859, Brisbane,
Queensland 4001, Australia

John Wiley & Sons (Canada) Ltd, 22 Worcester Road,
Rexdale, Ontario M9W 1L1, Canada

John Wiley & Sons (SEA) Pte Ltd, 37 Jalan Pemimpin #05-04,
Block B, Union Industrial Building, Singapore 2057

British Library Cataloguing in Publication Data

A catalogue record for this book is available from the British Library

ISBN 0-471-94001-1 (paper)

Typeset in 11/13 pt Times by Photo·graphics, Honiton, Devon
Printed and bound in Great Britain by Biddles Ltd, Guildford, Surrey

Contents

Series preface vii
Introduction ix
Acknowledgements x
Glossary of some Gestalt terms as used in this book xi
1 Sunday evening: Initial conditions 1
2 Monday morning: Survival 18
3 Monday afternoon: Insiders and outsiders 33
4 Monday evening: Thurber's war 46
5 Tuesday morning: The dream of leadership 59
6 Tuesday afternoon: Where do I belong? 73
7 Tuesday evening: The group beast 87
8 Wednesday morning: Dialogue 101
9 Wednesday afternoon: Pairing 117
10 Wednesday evening: Destructuring or destruction 131
11 Thursday morning: New configurations 144
12 Thursday afternoon: Nodal points and self-regulation 159
13 Friday morning: The group boundary 173
14 Friday afternoon: The wider gestalt 189
15 The follow-up: Assimilation, new awareness, and beginnings 202
Index 217

This book is dedicated to
Toby Owen, with love

Series preface

The Wiley Series in Psychotherapy and Counselling is designed to fulfil many different needs in advancing knowledge and practice in the helping professions. What unifies the books in this series is the importance attached to presenting clear authoritative accounts of theory, research, and experience in ways which will inform practice and understanding.

Gaie Houston has made a distinguished contribution to the development of group work through her previous publications, television broadcasts, consultancy activities, and contributions to professional training. This book represents a distillation of much of this experience in a form that is highly engaging and informative.

At the heart of this book lies the unending and puzzling struggle between the need that we all have for a sense of belonging and connectedness, and the need to be separate and individual. Gaie Houston brings new insights to this cyclic and vital process in a book which is bound to appeal to the widest lay and professional audience.

The author takes us through the intense experience of a five-day residential group in which the fictional participants represent Foulkesian, Kleinian, Systems, Psychodrama, Gestalt and other perspectives. The group members work their way through the week and battle to make clear the differences and commonalities between their theories. However, this is no ordinary account of theoretical debates about the nature of group dynamics. As the text makes clear all the participants feel the emotional reality of the deeply personal events they create. By means of this brilliant "drama-documentary" approach, the reader is drawn into this debate with a sense of urgency and involvement that can only be achieved through concrete "live" experience. Each chapter describes a morning, afternoon or evening in the life of the group and ends with a connecting commentary, that clarifies and integrates different perspectives in a way that is both original and un-dogmatic.

All those interested in group work who are willing to struggle with the attempt to understand what happens when people participate in experiential groups will find this book fascinating and deeply rewarding.

It is with great enthusiasm that this volume is welcomed to the series. It will prove to be an invaluable asset to group therapists and counsellors, and an inspiration to students.

John Allen
Series Editor

Introduction

Most people want to know more about themselves, and what makes them feel and behave the way they do with other people. That is the only prerequisite for reading this book. The glossary which follows the introduction may help readers unfamiliar with Gestalt terms to follow the more theoretical aspects of the events described.

Gestalt is commonly known as a therapeutic rationale and method. Group theory is not explicit within it, although most Gestalt training, and a good deal of the therapy, takes place in groups. So Gestalt practitioners use the findings of other schools to inform their work in groups. At the same time, many Gestalt concepts, especially those derived from Kurt Lewin, give fresh illumination to what goes on at group and systems levels, as well as personal and interpersonal levels. I hope this book makes clearer some few instances at least of the useful cross-fertilisation of theory.

The intensity of experience possible in small groups is not at all easy to convey. So, rather than talk at a general level, I have given an account of an imaginary residential group. My purpose is to give the reader a vivid impression of what may happen in such a setting.

None of the people attending the group described here are based on or represent specific individuals. Yet none of the people, the phenomena, the particular happenings and responses are merely fiction. In one or other of the many groups in which I have worked, people have gone through these kinds of experiences and developments. They have never in my presence so consistently and informedly talked over comparative theory. If they had, then there would perhaps have been less need for this piece of writing.

The explicit quest in this group meeting at Hartley Manor is set out in the first chapter. The implicit emotional quests of each person are also a strong part of their reality. The puzzling relation between the intensely personal and particular, and the cyclic and archetypal or near-inevitable, is perhaps what attracts readers to this subject. We want to make sense of ourselves and what we do. Labelling the understanding as belonging to this theory or that is to me of secondary interest. Belonging seems often, in a capitalist culture, to imply exclusivity, property, curtailment of freedom. Ian Mackrill kindly pointed out to me that I am not the only writer currently puzzling over a different sort of belonging—belonging as being connected to, allied with, formed by and forming the myriad groups that are in each life (Selby P., 1991, *Belonging—Challenge to a Tribal Church*. London: SPCK).

Having different participants write up each session is a reminder of how different the same people and events can seem to each member. Letting Jan, the group leader, add top and tail commentary to the chapters allows a connecting overview. That you, the reader, form yet another view and conclusion from the same evidence, is an outcome to be expected and welcomed. Gestalt is more to do with how we organise perception, than with what we are supposed to perceive.

Acknowledgements

The author is very grateful indeed to Toni Gilligan, Jane Puddy, John Leary-Joyce, Peggy Sherno, Jackie Clements, Nura Paul, Tina Pannell, Faye Page, Anna Farrow, Barrie Hinksman, Ian Mackrill, Eleanor O'Leary, Peter Bluckert, and Eva Coleman for their warmth and encouragement in this writing; to Adrian Mitchell for encouragement that has lasted forty years so far, as well as for permission to quote lines of his poems; to Malcolm Pines for his generous reading of the text and for his valued advice; to Jon Frew, Sonia March Nevis, Ruth Ronall, Bud Feder and Gary Yontef for the trouble they have taken to comment on various chapters and to hearten me from a Continent away.

Glossary of some Gestalt terms as used in this book

Aggression In Gestalt this word is used in its Latin meaning, to describe all outwardly directed activity.

Confluence Flowing together, with loss of boundary clarity. Healthy confluence is possible, as in *final contact (q.v.)*. Unhealthy confluence is a denial of contact-boundaries.

Contact-boundary Perls and Goodman were fascinated with the mutually constructed boundary between *organism*, usually meaning the self, and *environment*, often meaning the other person, as well as anything else. To them, this was the locus of awareness and experience.

Field A dynamic play of forces that forms a whole, perceived as a shifting *figure* against a *background*.

Figure What is foreground in awareness at any moment.

Formation, gestalt This is the configuring or organising process of moving from some disequilibrium of need, through to taking action (in Gestalt terms, aggressing), and then to withdrawal, and either gratification, or the learning that the action taken did not achieve what was needed. The four stages are:

1. *Fore-contact* The state of quest, unease, disequilibrium which leads to making a clear figure against a clear background. "Help, we've no table!" could be a simple fore-contact state for a home-buyer.

2. *Contact* From an internal state of fore-contact, attention goes to what is of interest in the world—in our example, the furniture shop. This is now the figure against a background of home-buying.

3. *Final contact* This is the probably brief merged state, when self recedes and the contact itself is highly figural. Orgasm is the most dramatic example of final contact. In the furniture shop example, the moment of seeing the table that "says something to you" is the equivalent. You let it into your life, perhaps buy it.

4. *Post-contact* When final contact has happened, there is withdrawal, learning, and then loss of interest in what was before so figural. The table, so carefully chosen and admired, becomes no more than a support for books and plates. Your attention is freed to attend to other things.

Gestalt There is no exact equivalent word for this German one. The meaning is to do with configuration, making a pattern. The underlying idea is that we constantly organise *fields* of data into *figures* or *foreground*, and *environment* or *background*. In a simple example, you may never have noticed furniture shops, until you thought of setting up home.

gestalt In this text, the word in lower case stands for a particular configuration. With a capital, it stands for the theory.

Introjection Swallowing whole, unchewed. This shorthand way of learning is useful in some instances, and highly dysfunctional in others.

Projection Seeing clearly in others attributes you may be much less aware of as being your own.

Retroflection Doing to yourself what you might want to do to others.

CHAPTER 1

Sunday evening: Initial conditions

"A GESTALT APPROACH TO THE GROUP"

"Gestalt practitioners, and professionals of other schools, are invited to a phenomenological exploration of group process. The form of the event will be planned by the participants and leader on the first evening. The leader, Jan Padrewski, is interested in integrating good practice from other schools into Gestalt group work, as well as in sharing his methods and present understanding of gestalting groups and larger systems (Beaumont 1990). He hopes for direct experiential learning, and as well, informed dialogue on different approaches. There is a good library at Hartley Manor. This will be an educational, not a therapy group."

Jan writes: That I, the leader of the group, would only learn about the first session of it from the notes of one of its members, was nowhere in the field when I wrote that advertisement so many months ago. Again I feel the despair of my interminable hours at Athens airport that day, imagining whether or how you would start. Ridiculously, I was in the grip of Bion's basic assumption, that everything was down to me, that only I, as parent–leader, could create the nurturing beginning. But there is fascination now for me in seeing what you did without me.

As I see it, some of my job was to fill out the background of theory, as we lived the actuality in our days of group life. So I have let myself add this comment, and more after Birde's notes. And I have added references as they occur to me.

I sat with my suitcase wedged under my legs, playing in imagination with how it was that this advertisement attracted you nine people, from so many countries and such diverse therapeutic disciplines, enough to make you pay up and turn up. You all must have been on certain mailing lists, or been primed in some way to bring to the foreground of your awareness advertisements of this kind. Your training probably accounts for that. And then we look at what accounts for your training. Genetics and upbringing; nature and nurture; chemistry and circumstances leading back generations may be the long paths that led each of you to this precision of synchronicity, to appear at this country house I remembered so clearly and so ruefully, on this summer's day. Ephemeral groups such as this are often called artificial. I see this one as profoundly organic.

This is the depth of field of this manifest group. In that depth are long acculturations in different places and nations. There are many political systems and assumptions about kinship obligations. As to many groups, each member arrived massively prejudiced, perhaps much more a stranger in a strange land than the homogeneity of summer T-shirts and jeans you all probably wore might suggest.

Traditions in the background

Let me justify calling you prejudiced. Birde's account of the first evening is coloured by her kind of training. Like many Gestalt practitioners, she has been educated to work one-to-one, in what can roughly be called the Perlsian tradition. Fritz, to many of you the best known originator of Gestalt therapy, kept some of the bias of the analytic tradition in which he was trained. Much of his therapeutic focus was on the intrapsychic and interpersonal. He gave less attention to the group as a psychic entity. Two-chair, or hot-seat, work was an excellent device which he developed and used extensively, for unscrambling The Great Muddle About Who Is Who (Houston 1982).

It was not until *Beyond the Hot Seat* (Feder and Ronall 1980) that a formal written attempt was begun to integrate knowledge

Initial conditions 3

of group dynamics into Gestalt therapy. The Cleveland Institute and the New York Gestalt Institute are among those who have done much to enlarge awareness of group within Gestalt. Many of their practitioners emphasise the building of safety and trust. From here have emerged what are termed Interactive Gestalt groups, in which the leader imposes a clear ethos of dialogue between members. In the traditional post-Perlsian group, more of the dialogue is likely to be between the leader and each member, so the leader can be seen as the hub of a wheel, with the members as spokes connecting first to him or her.

If I had been with you, I imagine I would have talked a little about Paul Goodman, the co-author (with Perls and Hefferline) of *Gestalt Therapy* Vol 2 (1951). His great interest was in societal issues. I believe that he was drawn to Gestalt partly as an attractive theory of group and social behaviour, as Goldstein and Lewin demonstrated (Goldstein 1939; Lewin 1951). Like these writers, like me, Birde has a sense I think of the group as a whole. But her training is in regarding the individual as the organism, with the group as its environment, perhaps. Implicitly she makes the group itself a figure in her account, on several occasions. But she has not yet the vocabulary to think what she feels.

Pierre's prejudice is to assume that the group is an entity. This is the polarity of Birde's and some other members' vision. No wonder Birde and Pierre clash. Practitioners like Pierre, influenced by Bion (1961), are likely to emphasise such issues as hostility and sexuality between group members and the conductor. At a first glance, this looks somewhat opposite to the safety and trust made salient in some Gestalt groups. At much the same time, Foulkes and Anthony (1957) were already concentrating on allowing free discussion rather than the free association that might be expected from the analytic school. They required value to be given to whatever might be said.

Manfred with his family therapy training stands for another way of looking at the group, as a system of interacting sub-groups, the behaviour of part expressing for and influencing the whole.

This first evening reminds me of a Foulkesian group, in its lack of imposed structure and norms. A massive difference, however, is that I, the central transferential figure as leader, *was not physically present*. But it looks as if I stayed figural all the same in the plethora of initial conditions. Except to Grace who knows me, it is obvious that I could only have had importance as a name and a role: that is the only existence I had for you, besides the reverberating presence of my absence.

Birde's account

Like a horse in its stable this ancient house stands quiet and content. We are fleas who leap here for a few days and then go or die. So many summers, so many people have happened here, and the house and garden have outlived them.

I sit at a table beneath a dormer window, with almost enough light from the growing moon to write by. An hour ago I lay down to sleep, tired out, but could not. The evening was so unfinished, so full and so full of gaps. I cannot let it go.

I arrived late because I missed the proper train from the airport. There was a lot of talking and laughing in the kitchen. I remember Chuck chasing Sohan, waving a tea towel. It took me some time to find that Jan was still not here. It was Annie who suggested we should meet in the library anyway. It does not look as if Jan can be here before tomorrow afternoon, so we decided on making written reports to help him see what has been going on.

I see now how smoothly and quietly I slipped in my offer to be the recorder for this evening, the moment Manfred asked if there was to be any note-taking for research. Good Gestalt would have been to remind people to take responsibility for themselves. Notes by everyone would make a far fuller account. The Nine Gospels.

I remember bits and pieces, not a clear sequence as I would like to. Who started? In a way it was Grace, saying, I think, that she was afraid she would be executed as the carrier of bad news when she told us that the air controllers' strike had kept Jan at Athens airport.

Like a spitting cobra, Sappho said that she had come from Greece today, by bothering to go to Thessaloniki and fly from there. Jan was a fool for not doing the same. There was much taking of sides, and showing of ourselves, I think: From me, "Poor Jan is American, so it is impossible that he has ever heard of any airport in Greece besides Athens." "Anyone can do anything if they really want to," from Manfred. "Perhaps," this from Orminda, "this is all part of his experimental method, and he is really spying

Initial conditions

on us from inside the massive chimneys, like the Securitate or something." Manfred said that idea was nonsensical, then went and looked up the chimney. The laughter was quite hysterical. When he talks, it is like linen tearing, violent, with many negatives, many verbs like deplore, object, fail.

Sohan, the young Indian, will be everyone's favourite. Or will the antipathy I have read of between Asians and West Indians mean that Grace is against him? I do not understand her. That must be my antipathy, I think. But in my small town in Sweden I have met few black people. I do not read her expressions. When she laughs I am sometimes startled. But she has trained in Gestalt in the States, so I have much to learn from her.

Drunk with travel-tiredness, I write what comes. Fantasy, id-processes, seem when I look back to have been the underground stream feeding our behaviour tonight. They are the prejudice and half-impressions and archaic fears that each member has, and that this one member is revealing.

Now I remember. Grace said that Jan was apologetic about the delay, and that he sent some advice. Chuck interrupted with something rather Australian about what Jan could do with his advice. Only now do I realise that we never heard what the advice was.

Annie was sorry for Jan. It is an awful thought that she is my age, I suppose. We are the older women of the group. I cannot bear it. Me so thin and she so fat, with such a bottom and belly under that great tent dress. That much fat must mean unhappiness. Unhappy therapists are not good.

It was Grace who pointed out that I was unhappy in the meeting, when I projected my unhappiness on to Jan. Now I project on Annie. So I remind myself that I am not doing what I hoped for with my life. I work too many hours only to pay my rent and my pension scheme. If I had stayed a social worker I would be provided for in so many ways. But the rebel in me makes me the independent one in a socialist country, so I am insecure, always short of money, sometimes hating my clients before I open the door to them. But not when I see them.

Sappho cut across an interesting observation I have forgotten, saying to Chuck, "Nobody really believes that Gestalt has any group theory of its own."

Sappho seems to take no notice of women, as if we are not

there, or are chairs to be pushed under the table as she waltzes towards the men. O yes, I am jealous. No, even this is not so baldly true. I am wistful to see such a perfect youthful creature. I would like black wavy hair to my waist, and a wonderful training in psychodrama as she has. I chose to ignore Sappho, and said mildly, "Please. In Gestalt each person speaks for herself only. You cannot know the group mood, Annie. I am sure you excuse that I correct you."

At once came the first intervention from Pierre. Pierre never chatters or laughs or discusses. Pierre makes interventions. I am sure also that he has a Liver, in the famous way of the French. He was quite angry with me for what I had said to Annie, which he told me I was really saying to Sappho: "There is a group mood; but Annie must not speak of it. *Sure you excuse that I correct you*! You know her feelings, then, and are allowed to speak for her? But she must not speak for others. This is absurd." He threw his hands in the air, then crossed his arms violently so his hands were hidden under his armpits, and pushed his chair back and closed his eyes.

"O, you are right. I blush. First I compete against Annie, then I try to placate (Satir 1972). Please tell me if I do such things again." This was a good Gestalt answer, open and undefensive and self-revealing. Pierre simply blew sharply through his nose, without opening his eyes.

There was a long silence, in which I thought of cutting things to say. I was ready to cry. I have borrowed money in order to be here. To work in groups with knowledge and skill is so much my ambition. And there I sat dumb among the dumb, appalled at my stupidity, and quite paralysed.

From bad to worse. The silence was broken, by Manfred saying coldly, "Nothing happens. I am considering leaving now."

This time Orminda was the rescuer, saying, "We are happening. We're the group who is going to study itself. I've trained with Carl Rogers (1970) and I trust the process. We ... sorry, Birde, I ... am discovering what we do now, and then we shall find how we cope with a late leader." I could have kissed her for being so sane and constructive.

Annie said, "A late leader. I got an image of a corpse. Carrying all the badness of the group for us." (Klein and Riviere 1952) She

Initial conditions

is a Kleinian, so everything is pre-Oedipal drama of Good and Bad, like an English pantomime, to her.

"I have much experience in groups. This group itself is of little value to me. It is Jan Padrewski I have come on an expensive journey to study with," said Manfred grandly. Orminda sounded desperate:

"My whole life is the journey that has brought me here. It has been expensive to me too. I want to learn from everyone. And one way to start would be for us at least to introduce ourselves. Can't we go round the circle?"

Pierre immediately said something cutting about the group search for a structure as a means of avoiding our murderous feelings. Orminda just said simply, "I am looking at all of you, struggling to recognise and be recognised (Schutz 1966) and to find a way to learn together."

After a time Grace voiced my feelings when she said, "My heart keeps sinking when we go silent again." So Pierre produced another of his From-Another-Planet remarks: "Something needs to be admitted in the group. There is the sense of a conspiracy to prevent this taboo being revealed."

"The great Gaul hath spoke. Let no dog ope his lips," said Grace, sounding furious. "Look, sonny, I have a doctorate in aspects of small and median group behaviour. You can take it from me, we're doing just fine. We know how to play the sensible grown-up who makes rational responses to what's happened to Jan. And we're letting out some of the irrational stuff, too (Bion 1961). So we are already working at the group task, and we've already got some consensus about how to do it: by expressing what is going on, rather than censoring." She is very able.

Now Pierre sounded rattled. "So is this the famous establishing of safety in the Gestalt group? It is an empty concept. The intention is evidently to hold the group in the primitive delusion that they have joined the family, the group, to receive nourishment and protection from the leader, and he will provide it" (Bion 1961, p. 147).

I found myself very defensive of Gestalt, and very stupid to find the flaws in what he was saying. Chuck said something about some beans at supper, farted, and said, "Sorry, folks. It's my unconscious uttering."

"By this gas emission you speak hostility to me, I think." said Pierre.

Grace made a good saving intervention. "I'm giggling like the others. And I'm listening to you as well, Pierre." All she got for her trouble was, "The caring Gestalt leader, who must always seduce. I cross myself against this," from Pierre. He did so.

Chuck smiled at her and said, "I liked your formulation about us being adult enough to be infantile, Grace. It kind of dignifies me. But I just felt mad. And I'd better come clean. Just because I'm a psychiatrist, please don't assume I know a damned thing about unconscious group processes and all. That's why I'm here, to learn. And if you people can teach me, then Jan can go stuff himself, as far as I'm concerned." Then little Sohan came in, and all of us smiled, welcoming him.

"I am a real charlatan, I assure you. I am called an art therapist, and I work with groups of patients in a psychiatric hospital. But I have only one year of training. I too need to learn. It is good to have solidarity with so highly qualified a participant."

"O boy. The blind leading the unsightly. Is there anyone besides old Manfred who's ever set foot in a group before? Come back, Jan, all is forgiven," said Chuck. I laughed. But I remembered too that Grace had spoken of her qualifications, and Chuck seemed to have forgotten this.

Manfred had got up and was taking books from a shelf in a way that annoyed me, and as it turned out, others. He suddenly read out, *"The career of a living system is nothing more than an organisational constancy measured against a backdrop of internal and external perturbations"* (Efran, Lukens and Lukens 1990).

Orminda suggested the Gestalt idea that we might learn more from the present than from books. Grace spoke of the hostility to Gestalt that kept surfacing. Orminda said something like, "I know what Pierre is likely to say back about inevitable conflict, and the release of energy in expressed hostility. But please let us live here in peace." She looked so vulnerable. But Pierre still intoned, "The image of not-peace, of murder, returns."

Orminda almost screamed at him, "Shut up! Just shut up your clever above-it-all interpretations!" She looked shocked at herself, and quickly added, "I'm sorry."

Suddenly Manfred put down his book and stood and spoke helpfully. I was so grateful! I so needed someone to take over. He put an empty chair forward, saying it was the key to our difficulties. I stared, fearing that the chair represented Gestalt, which seemed such a dirty word here. Someone told Manfred to go ahead and family-therap us. So Sappho objected that this was a Gestalt group, not a family therapy one. I offered that Gestalt is about raising awareness, assimilating and integrating, so I supported Manfred. Somehow he needs protection, though he is so superior.

But Sappho parroted Pierre's attitude to Gestalt, shouting, "All therapy is about raising awareness! I am not here to be told that psychodrama I learned directly in the Moreno Institute is really Gestalt all the time. Already Perls stole from Moreno. Now Gestalt is to devour systems theory and psychoanalysis and then say it is all Gestalt!" Manfred addressed her, I think by mistake, as Sophia. She spat at him, right in his face. He suggested that she was putting herself in a solitary place of opposition. About then Grace came in using that low easy voice of hers, making things seem more normal. Nanny was in the nursery and we were good children suddenly.

"Talk about first skirmishes! (Bennis and Shepard 1978) I'll join you in the lions' den for a couple of minutes, Manfred. Come on, get up, everybody. Look, rather than go on talking, let's just display our positions. If you're right behind Sappho, go there. If you're alongside Manfred, stand beside him. If you're vacillating, walk between them. If you turn your back on the whole thing, do so. You're getting the idea faster than I can spell it out. Just make figures of speech into action, so we see what we mean without using so many words. Change your position when you change your mind."

It was a relief to move about, showing where we stood in this literal way. Sappho quickly changed from her solitary position to stand between Pierre and Chuck, hugging them somewhat sexually. I think. We talked all at once, but also listened.

When he could make himself heard, Manfred asked where we were to put the chair, which he said symbolised where Jan was sitting. Chuck suggested out of the window. I got us to stand in a circle with our arms round each other, and said that when Jan came, I wanted him in an equal place with all of us.

Of course Pierre pulled away from the comforting circle and walked about saying, "But he is not the same as us! This is the egalitarian myth. There would not be gods, there would not be monarchies, unless there was a strong urge within groups to create leaders. And destroy them. You want to short-circuit a painful process, for the sake of this dream of peace. Nirvana at the price of honesty."

Manfred replied quietly, "So in this passionate disagreement the search is for an agreed structure for this family. The central task you have so quickly arrived at is this. There is concern for the absent leader, and there is recognition of the abilities of all the other family members. Perhaps you are saying that you are not just the babies in the nursery waiting for Papa. You are the grown-up children returned, who must find out what you all have learned on your journeys."

At this point Sohan sat on the chair, which was in the middle. He said that he wanted to show that he felt smaller than the rest of us, like a child. Annie suggested that we all sit down, and too that we finish soon. We had not agreed a stopping time. Manfred said, "So we have discovered that Padrewski's absence is our problem. And now we are searching for a structure which will take the place of a person as leader."

Much wrangling. I remember Chuck saying, "Strewth. You and Pierre. It's like living at Delphi or somewhere. The oracles. I give you notice, mate. I don't like it. I don't like feeling about three years old, and having you talk down to me." I had a sudden image I shared with the group.

I remembered the English book about the boy who receives his education from the magician Merlin, by becoming in turn many animals (White 1939). This experience integrated in him so he became a whole that is greater than the sum of the parts. I felt we could be Manfred's sick family, Sohan's art class, Sappho's psychodrama, and so on, and so enrich our own theories. I think even Pierre was co-operative, not agreeing directly, but asking for a seminar time each day. Sappho began to flirt with him, and Chuck joined in. It was a little nauseating. Thankfully Grace butted in, "Hey, I'd like to hear from everyone about taking turns being facilitator or therapist. We're doing just what Jan suggested, planning a form for the whole event on the first evening." I think she said something about it being too good to be true. She also asked if Manfred would tell us some theory straightaway.

Again Annie said how tired she was. But Manfred ploughed on as if she had not spoken. "The first necessity was that I join the family, to gain your confidence, to make rapport. I then ask myself:

Initial conditions

what is the problem in this family? With this question goes the important corollary: What is the function of the problem in the system? (Minuchin 1977) It was clear that the missing father was made the problem. What this perhaps did was to mask the struggle for leadership within the family. Birde's scheme of a clear rotation has satisfied the underlying need. My task was to see the family as a system, striving for some sort of balance in order to function. By positively connoting the present behaviours, I raised the self-esteem of the family. My positive re-framing of what could be destructive interactions allowed development to Birde's solution, and consensus (Gustafson and Cooper 1990). This is a great progress." Annie said that she had not heard any of it. I took notes, or I would not have remembered a word.

Pierre now leapt across to the bookcase and read out, *"It matters less what the therapist is selling than what the patient is buying. In the long run, people buy true, and that is what works. It is a mistake to think that the right re-framing statement transforms experience— not for long it doesn't"* (Nichols 1987).

Except when he was playing family therapist, Manfred is just awful; but I pitied him as Pierre slammed the book shut and smirked. I do not know if the group can support two such arrogant people as him and Pierre.

Sappho interrupted in her strange English, "Talk! I hear of nothing but talk. It is not hygienic, I mean it is not healthy, to sit and sit and be upset and then be clever. I need to move and express in all modalities, of mime and dance and song and painting."

Poor Annie said something about there being so many threads in our talk, and wondering if we would ever make a pattern of them. I did my best to build on what she said, by saying I did not yet have a sense of what thread she represents, or Grace, or Pierre. How co-operative I sounded! But I think I was making sure I was more powerful than her. Annie said something like, "I feel a bit of a lost soul, Birde. I'm divorced, so I have my children part of the time, and then I'm alone and lonely. I'm trained as a Kleinian psychotherapist. But recently I've started wanting to move on. To working with groups, maybe. But maybe wanting to quit my training is like the wanting to quit my husband. I just don't know."

I thought how I want to move on from the repeated miracles of Gestalt hot-seat work, to more understanding of all these frightening group dynamics. But I kept quiet and let Grace speak.

"I've got three kids. By three different fathers. I'm in an on-off sort of a relationship with my partner now. I do Gestalt training, and a lot of supervision and two therapy groups and some one-to-one counselling. I get tired thinking of it. I take too much responsibility, yes. I'd like to give that up here. And more than that, I want us this week to make some contribution to Gestalt group theory that is useful to anyone, not just professional Gestaltists."

In his completely egocentric way, Pierre said that there was too much hostility in the group, so he would resist what he called the group pressure to reveal himself. Chuck came right back at him, "My Grandad used to say, 'No smell till you got here'. Speak for yourself, mate. I feel hostile as hell towards you, and that's for sure."

In me there were such conflicts. Most urgently I want this group to be successful. And I have a fear of it falling to pieces already.

I let myself do something I know I am strangely good at, and I told Pierre's story, though I have never met him before. To do it, I had to be the best of myself, rather than this angry jealous person I could so easily be here. Now I reflect that perhaps that was what Manfred had done for a short time when he helped the group.

I told, "You are an eldest child, Pierre. You have younger sisters, two at least, but no brothers. You were always a very clever boy. In the family you get your own way very much, and you are copying your father, who tyrannises a little on your mother. Yes, you are married, I think. I back off this subject. I think you lived always in your family of origin or your married family. Under this bluster you are very shy. But. You have no children, or one child?"

All he said was, "Part of the group wishes to place me on this empty chair of leadership." Dear Sohan asked if what I had said was true; but Pierre just looked at the wall and said he had a strong sense of being manipulated.

Chuck was suddenly my prince on a white charger, and called Pierre a four-star pratt. Another row started, and I interrupted, my hands trembling, with a ridiculous sense that something, I know not what, perhaps my sanity, or Gestalt, or reality itself, must be saved. I gave a summing up, by asking people to stand, and sculpting my present vision of us as a group.

I put Pierre at the centre, like a strange witch-doctor in a frightened village. Grace was the calm mother; Chuck I had walking

Initial conditions 13

round, with his feet firmly on the ground, laughing and giving perspective. Sohan I put sitting near Chuck, secure as the group child. Sappho I asked to bounce among us like a rubber ball. Manfred I had making one sure-footed approach, then going right outside to the edges of the room. Annie I saw floating, seeing misty visions of us, while I pushed with one elbow to come in and take over. Orminda had to hold out her arms to try to contain us all, then sink back into herself, despairing.

I felt resentful when at the end of this, Annie only said again that she wanted to go to bed. She asked us to make clear time-boundaries tomorrow. She was getting at me, I think. Grace smiled and said it was bedtime, and everyone got up.

Jan's comment

Wow. What a lot there was to fight over. And how you went to it! All you guys had signed up to a Gestalt group, and you start by having a good scrap with Gestalt itself. Or maybe with me as well? And you got through so much work, though Birde does not seem to notice the successes of the evening.

Wilfred Bion wrote his brilliant description of the group as having two modes, ten years after *Gestalt Therapy* (Perls, Hefferline and Goodman, 1951). A Gestalt translation of this idea is that there are two poles. One is the timeless primitive basic assumption group, always accessible in the emotional life of the group. The other is the work group, which has structure, and allows the individuation of members. I find myself with this notion a lot of the time as I read this report. What is expressed sometimes as arguments over theories or methods, also smells to me of a more panicky fight and flight mode which is below all this ego stuff. Do understand me. What I call the ego, the rational disputes, have value in themselves. But at moments you shouted and even spat, in ways reminiscent of the nursery. There was a lot of feeling.

Now, a great strength of Gestalt is its emphasis on the obvious. Like Zen teachers, Gestaltists prefer often to cultivate the top three inches, rather than dig and dig and perhaps despoil the landscape. Perls had not much truck with the idea of the unconscious as a topological entity, though he set himself to

...investigate the theory and method of creative awareness, of figure/background formation, as the coherent center of the powerful but scattered insights into the 'unconscious' and the inadequate notion of the 'conscious'.

So I suggest that Bion provides some amplification of theory for Perls and for Gestalt. I speculate that you were in part fighting for survival, and maybe terrified of being overwhelmed or at the other pole, being excluded. Fight and flight, taking control and leaving, recur as themes. But, I bet you kept telling yourselves, we are all adult, and know how to run groups. We should manage this hiatus of formal leadership perfectly well. What is more, most of you, most of your working lives, labour to encourage members of your groups into some level of independence, of autonomy or inter-dependence—of something other than gross dependence. Yet here you were, flailing round like scared, hostile, total beginners.

The Gestalt reality is that you were complete beginners. You had never been in this house, this task, this group together before. And what is more, I had let you down.

Birde was very active, taking responsibility for events. The idea came to me once more as I read her words, that in her mind and the minds of all the rest of you, *the group already existed by the time you all sat down*. Sappho and Manfred seem as if they have farted in church when they speak of leaving. I imagine them knowing, somehow or other, that there is a boundary round a new entity, this group. They *belong* to it, willy-nilly. Orminda and others work to make the space within the boundary a good one to live in. But it is too soon. Too much adjustment to the new, almost to the sentence of being condemned to the group, still needs to happen.

Perhaps each person is constructing an imaginary boundary round this collection of strangers, and attempting to fill it with the pattern of group behaviour he or she somehow expects. Unless Orminda can make her Rogerian group, she may have to become a fighter. If Pierre cannot hold the group as an example of unconscious group process, his competence is out of the window. I suggest these comparatively superficial adjustments or losses. Without doubt there are more profound and archaic losses of familiarity threatened in any such permutation of human beings. The group looks a possible haven to some members, and more of a threat to others.

But as far as I can see, you were fighting a rearguard action. *The question was not the apparent one, of whether the group is to exist. It is only a question of how it is to exist, and how therefore it is to enhance or limit the nine of you already caught in its net.* Those human tendencies summed up in the Law of Praegnanz, towards simplifying, evoking, completing, have created the group as figure, against a jumble of competing personal fields.

Or perhaps something different is happening: *each is becoming a strand in the emergent self of the collective* (Stern 1985). Saying this, I think of a confluence of individuals into a different whole. In the last paragraph I described what may be an easier idea for you to take on board: a tournament of individual myths about the kind and character of the emerging group. It takes a moment to feel the difference, specially the emotional difference, between these possibilities. I often guess that, out of awareness, group members are struggling with this very conundrum. And I imagine that you will go on doing so through the week.

Yet another way of saying these two ideas is by asking: Do the individuals form the group, or does the group form the individuals in it? I very much hope that, however drawn you are to one, and scornful of the other notion, you will not take sides too quickly.

Leland Bradford used to say comfortingly that there is far more data generated in any group than can ever be processed. There is work for a year for us all in just this session.

What on earth advice did I, in my own panic, send you by telephone? I have forgotten, and you were never told. You elected to go it alone, and seemed to me to set about a perilous and brave journey.

The fights over methods echo to me as if they are fights between psyches struggling to survive, let alone become dominant in the Lewinian field of the group. A major struggle seems to me to have been, as in many groups, about whether a power system or an intimacy system is being agreed. Either involves denial of some of the needs of each member. Perls insisted tirelessly that aggression, in the sense he used the word, is part of intimacy. I notice as I read that that belief did not seem to be strong in you. Orminda calls openly for peace. Pierre mutters of murder, annihilation. These are the epic themes I see in group after group. And you are allowing them near the surface, attended by inevitable fear, foreboding and near-despair, at the very first meeting. Bennis and Shepard (1978) refer to the anxiety-avoiding behaviour that can happen early in a group. I imagine it there in the seeming neatness of the T.H. White plan. Otherwise it was not much in evidence.

Now and fore-contact

Birde's account shows the depth and extraordinary complexity of this moment, now, as you all experienced what Perls (1951) calls the fore-contact phase. This phase is informed by each person's own history, by their expectations, and by the impact of each on the other in the present. There is an almost exponential increase in complexity of fore-contact as the numbers in what is deemed to be a small group increase. A small group I define here as one of up to about fifteen people, in which there is time, even if not energy, for face-to-face contact in which the members can come to be known to each other with some understanding.

Agreeing what to do and how to do it is a simple description of what is emotionally here a titanic struggle to establish a Lewinian field, or what I call a large gestalt, a shared reality and purpose which leads to a series of acceptable gestalt formations within it.

Even within this turmoil of over-stimulus, a temporal completion is achieved. Implicit in Birde's wish to bring everyone into the group is the sense that this gestalt will influence the forming of tomorrow's. Agreement on a small gestalt suggests that the overarching one is emerging from the shadows.

References

Beaumont H. (1990) Unpublished lecture to the Gestalt Centre, London. Hunter Beaumont uses the word *gestalt* as a verb as well as a noun, to give a sense of the constant becoming.

Bennis W. and Shepard H. (1978) A theory of group development. In: L. Bradford (Ed.), *Group Development*, La Jolla: University Associates.

Bion W. (1961) *Experiences in Groups.* London: Tavistock Publications, pp. 143–147.

Bradford L.P., Gibb J.R. and Benne K.D. (1964) *T-Group Theory and Laboratory Method.* New York: John Wiley.

Efran J., Lukens M. and Lukens R. (1990) *Language, Structure and Change.* New York: W. W. Norton, p. 47.

Feder B. and Ronall R. (1980) *Beyond the Hot Seat—A Gestalt Approach to Group*. New York: Brunner-Mazel.
Foulkes S.H. and Anthony E.J. (1957) *Group Psychotherapy—The Psycho-Analytic Approach*. Harmondsworth: Penguin.
Gleick J. (1988) *Chaos: Making a New Science*. London: Heinemann.
Goldstein K. (1939) *The Organism*. Boston: American Book Co.
Gustafson J.P. and Cooper L.W. (1990) *The Modern Contest*. New York: W.W. Norton, pp. 21–22.
Houston G. (1982) *The Red Book of Gestalt*. London: Rochester Foundation, pp. 83–89.
Klein M. and Riviere J. (Eds) (1952) *Developments in Psycho-Analysis*. London: Hogarth Press.
Lewin K. (1951) *Field Theory in Social Science*. New York: Harper and Brothers.
Minuchin S. (1977) *Families and Family Therapy*. London: Tavistock.
Nichols M.P. (1987) *The Self in the System*. New York: Brunner-Mazel.
Perls F., Hefferline R. and Goodman P. (1951) *Gestalt Therapy. Excitement and Growth in the Human Personality*. New York: Julian Press.
Rogers C. (1970) *Carl Rogers on Encounter Groups*. New York: Harper and Row, p. 51.
> One of his great contributions was his constant valuing of the authority of each person about herself. He came to dream of the possibility of global harmony, achieved in part through the work of large groups, which would respect and listen to all their members, and so find their own wisdom and better ways to live. It is easy to smile at such idealism. Perhaps it is an indicator of possibilities.

Satir V. (1972) *Peoplemaking*. Palo Alto: Science and Behaviour Books.
Schutz W.C. (1966) *The Interpersonal Underworld*. Palo Alto Science and Behaviour Books.
> Schutz postulates only three sorts of behaviour in groups. Members work at: *Inclusion*, by which he meant recognition, acceptance and their opposites; *Control*, everything to do with action and decision-making, and *Affection*, by which he meant the full gamut of pairing activity.

Simkin J. and Yontef G. (1984) Gestalt therapy. In: R. Corsini (Ed.) *Current Psychotherapies*. Ithaca: Peacock.
Stern D. (1985) *The Interpersonal World of the Infant*. New York: Basic Books.
White T.H. (1939) *The Sword in the Stone*. London. Hart-Davis.
Yontef G. (1980) *Gestalt Therapy: A Dialogic Method*. Unpublished paper, privately circulated.
Zinker J. (1977) *Creative Process in Gestalt Therapy*. New York. Brunner-Mazel.

Chapter 2

Monday morning: Survival

Jan writes: At moments I felt my hair bristle up the back of my neck with fear as I read Grace's account. Dimly, I saw psychic survival as the primary task. John Frew calls this the Orientation stage of forming a group (Frew 1992).

Is it rivalry or is it parenting that makes me want to list one or two descriptions by different schools, of this stage of group life? To hell with the motivation; let's get on with the behaviour.

Adler (1929) would argue that you are competing, because of issues of status. You are skirmishing about a pecking order. This hypothesis is out of fashion in much of Western culture at the moment. Equal opportunities, democracy, are not ideas which sit easily for many with the notion of a constant hierarchical striving.

Schutz (1966) might argue that some of the behaviour in the group is to do with belonging, with Inclusion. People are struggling with questions like:

> Will they let me in?
> Do I want to join?
> Do I feel like letting him or her in?

Anzieu (1984) might stress at this point the tension between hostility between members, and the fear of fragmentation of the group.

Other theorists see the amount of competition likely between members of this group. You are working, sometimes by rival methods, perhaps all with a sense of being under-informed, in the same area. You can show yourselves up, and show each other up (Goffman 1967; Durkin 1981). This is, I think, the fear that shows in Birde's and Grace's accounts.

Self

Each of these briefly-mentioned theories is to do with survival. They are about the survival of the sense of self. In Gestalt the self only finds and makes itself in the environment. According to Perls (1951):

> ...the self is precisely the integrator: it is the synthetic unity, as Kant said. It is the artist of life. It is only a small factor in the total organism/environment interactions, but it plays the crucial role of finding and making the meanings we live by (p. 235).
>
> The self is not to be thought of as a fixed institution; it exists wherever and whenever there is in fact a boundary interaction ... Self, the system of contacts, always integrates perceptive proprioceptive functions, motor-muscular functions and organic needs (p. 373).

The survival of each member's self-esteem is linked to the survival or destruction of the group. Is belonging to this group to be added to the identity of each person here, as part of their process of excitement and growth? Freud (1922) postulated the primal horde, who killed and cut up the father, then banded together as an equal brotherhood. From this, he suggested, the myth of the hero came, as one person—perhaps the youngest brother as in so many fairy-stories—was credited with the manliness of standing up against authority. In this powerful speculation, Freud saw this as the emergence of the individual from group psychology. In other words, he alleges that group identity or consciousness predates individual perception. Sullivan (1950) also spoke of the delusion of unique individuality. The profoundly disturbing theme of individual *versus* group identity is mostly implicit rather than explicit in Grace's report. Her relation to me seems one of the self-esteem or survival constructs in her mind (Kelly 1955).

Grace's account

Well, I did the whole earth-mother ain't-she-just-wonderful number again this morning. Damn.

Do you remember, Jan, how we used to walk along the beach at Key Largo, saying in our best imitations of upper-class English, "Tell me, Colonel, what is your opinion of the feeling of the meeting this morning?" The feeling of the start of this meeting, brother, was death by depression masked by death by pretence. Sappho's short-wave radio helped her come in late, spend real time dragging chairs around and exchanging cushions with unwilling partners, before announcing that the strike at Athens was continuing, so she knew absolutely that you would not be here till tomorrow at the earliest.

Silence. Manfred white as a sheet and studying the linenfold panelling, as he did most of the morning. Orminda white as a sheet, slowly wringing her hands, and darting anxious little looks at everybody when she thought they were not looking at her.

Pierre sat with his hands on his knees, being a group conductor: smug behind an invisible glass screen. Birde kept smiling brightly at people. Annie seemed a dead loss, a great bulging sack of gloom in the best armchair. Until I started writing, I did not know how angry I was with them.

Before Sappho threw her stink-bomb, Chuck had begun the group:

"At the end of last night's meeting in here I was in need of six strong men and a wheelbarrow to get me to bed. Then Annie started pointing out all these stars I didn't know. I was bright as a button again. And now I feel as heavy as hell, coming back in here this morning." Birde did one of her warm concerned explore-the-feeling replies. I bet myself she'd start talking about this being a Healing Group before the day was out. Her tolerance of conflict is around nil.

There's a funny feeling in my head, as if I'm skipping past a lot, pushing away a lot that is really there in me. Pause. What I feel as if I'm doing is ganging up on them. Gang up with you. So I sort of acknowledge my bias, more than I like to admit, and push on regardless.

Chuck, who really does look like one of the very healthy people, started to show himself. "Maybe I didn't come clean last night.

I've got a hell of a lot of scepticism about whether therapy in groups, or life in groups, come to think of it, has anything going for it whatsoever."

At this point Orminda said in a desperate tone, "How about moving into the garden? It's a beautiful day." Pierre did pipe up at this:

"I fear that changing locations will be another avoidance." I told him he sounded like Jeeves with a French accent. As he and most of them had never heard of P.G. Wodehouse, this went down like a lead balloon. Maybe you haven't. Hell. I may be black, but I am British, you know. Jan, I am kind of horrified at all this jokiness in me, specially when you see what a lot of the morning was about. It's just the mood I get into, remembering the first part.

Paralysis followed for a while, tinged for me at least with blackest doom. Annie asked Pierre what he thought we were avoiding. No. I'm muddled about the start. Beginnings of groups exhaust me.

"Hic et nunc. What is here and now," said Pierre, in those toffee-nosed tones I loathe so much. Little Twinkletoes Birde put her wee head on one side and gasped, "But that's amazing! An analyst talking Gestalt."

Incapable of taking a compliment, Pierre snapped that he was not an analyst. "I am a lecturer in clinical psychology. Of course I apply analytic perspectives. I have experience of Foulkesian group methods. And the here and now is a fundamental of that method, above all in the group. The group is the place of diagnosis in the present. And for me part of the present is my dilemma of role. Am I a participant, with the duty of full disclosure of what goes on in my consciousness? Or am I a monitor, an observer, a therapist, staff member, who is abstinent, but not necessarily disclosing?" To this Birde lisps prettily, "This is a Gestalt group. I want to be me here. And I want you to be you."

I have calmed down a bit now. What came next? Sappho again, I think, saying, "Jan betrays us. I did not sleep, almost not at all. And I think seriously I shall leave now and refuse to pay the rest of my money." Annie said, "I notice how profoundly it upsets me to hear you say that. As if we shall be destroyed if you go. I felt real anger at you for saying it. Just for a second."

"This is a sort of blackmail. I refuse it!" said Sappho. Annie heaved out of the depths of her obesity to say Sappho was projecting all that was ugly and bad in her on to the group, and that Annie for one could not stand it. Or something like that. Sappho retorted something that seemed a verbal version of sticking her tongue out. Orminda pulled her feet back under her chair and twisted her hands harder. Chuck flung about in his chair. Birde threw in something really wet about women being sisters. Yuk yuk.

I am rivalling Birde to be Female Gestalt Queen in this group.

You say that structures obscure organic process. I say that structures can channel process without stopping its flow. Anyway, since you were not here, and I was, I offered to put in some Gestalt, and saw nods from all but Manfred, who afterwards denied that he had not agreed, and then would not agree, but only shrug. A killjoy. At this stage I saw him and Annie and Sappho as the worst potential trouble in the group.

I think I did a short input about awareness. Without awareness of each other's feelings and inner world, we would live a delusion. Looking back, I see that as a Benne and Sheats (1948) intervention. Using their categories, I was apparently dealing with individual needs, which were obviously to do with the group task of looking at the group, and which had a clear group building intention as well.

Manfred winked at Pierre, whom he certainly needs as his ally, and said, "These Gestaltists have a strange belief in the power of biography." Pierre merely returned a toad-like stare. I suppressed a wish to grab hold of either of them by his hair the way my Jamaican grandmother would have done. She'd have bent him over and run him round the kitchen, shouting at him to speak to her CIVIL! Then she'd've shoved him out of the back door, telling him not to show his face around here again until he'd learned some manners. But I am so boringly white nowadays, I just explained how many different meanings Manfred might attribute to the look, unless Pierre revealed more, probably in words. Earnest nodding from Sohan, Birde, Orminda. A slight head inclination from Annie, a grunt from Chuck. Sappho got up and sat between Pierre and Manfred, both of whom, I swear it, were mad with delight at capturing her.

My heart was in my boots. By the time you get here, it looks as if we shall be habituated to behaving as a basic assumption group (Bion 1961).

I feel quite proud of myself that I have written a moment-to-moment account, without hinting at what came next. The transition was so abrupt. The group transformed from snakes, or maybe tigers or jackals, to being therapists, which I suppose for many of us is the best way we know how to be.

Somebody, I think it was Annie, cut across Chuck starting to swear at the other men, and pointed out that Orminda was in tears. She was sitting alongside me, so I had not noticed. No. She was sitting alongside me AND I had not noticed that tears were streaming down her face (Perls 1971, for examples of attention to use of words). Her mouth was grimacing, as if she was working to keep it from trembling. But there were no sobs. There was something very alarming about her, which everyone must have recognised. We waited for her, and when she said she could not bear to be looked at, Pierre spoke very gently to the rest of us about the transformation in his feelings when he saw Orminda's distress. Quiet agreement from many. We knew what we were doing—being with Orminda, without intruding her. And we were getting on with the task. If there was a scanner on group morale, I think the line would have gone up almost vertically at this point, from its all-time low a minute before.

After a while I adapted some of what I had said about awareness, inviting Orminda to talk if she wanted to. Annie said something like, "Orminda, I have a strong impression that you are doing something quite violent to yourself." Orminda wrung her hands more, and said, "If I start I shall just take up too much time and I don't even need to. I can cope."

Birde spoke quietly; "Orminda, I see how skilled you are to turn the conversation away from you. Annie asks you of your sad looks." Birde has great presence at such moments. I imagine she is an excellent one-to-one therapist. But even at this moment our insecure ugly lad, Manfred, could not forbear picking a fight, saying coldly, "To call her sad is an interpretation. And everywhere I read that Gestalt forbids absolutely the interpretation. Please answer this. I have strongly the feeling that I have studied more the depth of Gestalt from its philosophical origins than have others." Unforgivable, at this moment. Orminda was sitting there with this air of devastation, and being ignored.

Annie spoke then. I could somehow float with the feel of her image. But my hair actually stood on end. I felt it.

"We, you, are burying hearts in dark earth. We can cope. The group is to cope by being ego-centred, by operating from above the shoulders." Birde focussed us back on Orminda, in a less obscure way. She and Annie make a good team.

"Orminda, you have heard us. And I see how affected you are. I want you to know that I can cope too if you don't want us to know what is troubling you. Of course I shall be unquiet; but that is a problem for me. I do not want to coerce you." A decent dialogic response. Orminda grasped at it: "But I don't want anybody's sympathy! I can really do without that." I did a knee-jerk response: "So I've heard what you don't want. What DO you want?" "I want to stop sobbing," she said. Though she hardly was. The sobs seemed to be stopped way down in her solar plexus. Now we were into one-to-one, in the way you deplore in a group setting. I guess I wanted to keep Manfred and Sappho, even poor Sohan, from trampling all over Orminda. It is quite hard to convey the feeling of urgency, of disaster, that I was sensing. So I said, "I want us to slow down, and stay with your not-coping as well as your coping. I know I want to be quiet for a while."

There was a long silence, broken by Orminda. She spoke more or less as I quote her, in her soft Irish accent.

"Thanks for the tissues. There's bits of this story I've never told and I need to. I don't want sympathy. I've had a year and two weeks of lugubrious hypocritical sympathy.

I'm from a Catholic family in Cork. And when I was working in Scotland I met Michael. He was a Protestant from Belfast. That was four years ago. We were working on a project, taking Rogerian methods into sixteen schools. I was running it."

Birde said it sounded as if she was telling the story for us, and asked if Orminda could find a way to tell the story for herself, at the same time as being aware that she was offering it to us. She seemed to take this in, and when she went on, was less tense and effortful.

"God, was I the cock of the walk! Didn't the sun just shine out of my arse-hole? The children responded; the teachers ate out of our hands; Michael said he was in love with me. And then he got the invitation to take the same kind of Rogerian method into all the schools of a little town outside Belfast. It seemed meant, in a crazy grandiose way. Michael and I would be married and symbolise the re-unification of Ireland, and electrify the entire educational system of Europe, given a couple of years. So we got married all

Survival

in a rush without even meeting each other's parents. Ignoring the background, you'd maybe call it in Gestalt. And then we went to his little town and met his widowed mother." She stopped herself, saying she was going on too long. Patient interventions from Annie and Chuck. She steadied herself and went on:

"The centre of it is, it was a poor thin kind of a marriage. And when Siobhan was born two years ago, her left foot was withered, the leg a bit short. I can't help crying again; but it's all right. She learned to put her teddy under her foot when she pulled herself up to stand."

It was terrible to hear. Now look, I have a nephew with a club foot. I did that project I told you about, with parents of dying children. But today I could hardly bear to hear of such an unjust, such a wanton affliction on a baby. Sappho cried quietly, Annie shrank into tears, and I feared she would start yelling silently for attention. You know me, I was crying too. Birde kept us going, saying to Orminda, "You are coping again. You are pushing past your feelings to make the story clear for us. Please, tell the story for you, to hear yourself."

"Yes." She went quiet before starting up again, "Just over a year ago she was fretful one evening, and I brought her downstairs. I had a dressing gown with a hood, and she went quiet always if she could creep her head into the hood, and lean on my shoulder. Then Michael wanted supper, and wanted me to get it. We kind of wrangled about it. In the end he draped the dressing gown round his head and took Siobhan and sat in front of the telly. I went to the kitchen. Then there were the shots."

Another silence. No helpful interventions, no distraction. We all looked as if we had been shot, I think. I had begun to dread a bomb story. Living in America, you probably don't know about these almost daily news items of car-bombs in Northern Ireland, death by explosion and fragmentation, so often of fathers of young families. So often followed by an apology from the IRA or the UDA for an unfortunate mistake in their choice of victim. Followed by a revenge killing the next day or week. And on. Orminda's voice came into the quiet. Maybe she didn't stop speaking, and the silence was just a blast in my head.

"Both of them were there on the floor. They both were alive another few minutes. The bit of the story I've never uttered is that some time, even before the police got there, I think, a neighbour came in and told me that Michael's mother had shot herself. And I said it must have been that she was so upset to learn of the deaths. I said I'd phoned her. But I hadn't.

She shot him. I knew it straightaway. She shot him thinking it was me in that dressing gown, and then saw what she'd done."

Annie said softly that it was like a Greek tragedy. Sappho tried to ask something about the police, and I interrupted, like the autocrat you have called me:

"These questions are not at the centre of this story. Three deaths and all Orminda's feelings about them are the centre." I was right, Jan. Because Pierre immediately opened his mouth. I'm pleased to say that Chuck immediately delivered him a verbal uppercut:

"Orminda asked for peace." Amazingly, Pierre looked back at him and half-flushed, just up his neck as far as his mouth, and said, "I apologise. I'm ashamed. The story is too dreadful. She forbids sympathy. But embracing her is the group need."

"Yes. Orminda. An O of arms round you is the image that keeps coming into my mind," said Annie. Orminda asked if she could go over and sit with Annie and be held by her, because she looked so soft.

"I look fat. Let me come to you. Manfred, will you move, please?"

"I'm so horribly bony. A bony little girl. Yes, you just holding me is everything. It's the first time." Orminda settled against Annie, who held her quietly, while she sat and shook and then gradually relaxed. Birde commented that it was the first time for a long time, perhaps, that Orminda had let herself stop coping. The task was to give value to Orminda, a group member who looks self-depriving, bewildered, in some kind of post-traumatic shock. I know damn well that I could have used a group-involving method to do it. I could have let well alone. I could have asked Orminda if she would like to hear back from other people in the group. But no, off I went with a perfectly functional intervention; it was just one that corralled the protagonist into my care. I said:

"You told us this strange part of the story, of your suspicions of Michael's mother, and your cover-up. Notice what is different for you now that we know this secret. It is not a secret now." Oh well, maybe I was hard on myself. That is a bit group-oriented. Orminda sounded authentic, all there, as she answered:

"I feel as if I've arrived. Transparent, and very tired, and relieved. I can see you holding back on sympathy statements, and I'm grateful. I don't mind you talking more about all this. But for me, that can be outside group time. I need to rest now. Carry on as if I'm not here. I'll soon interrupt if I need to." I wanted her to know that she had authority in the group. And I wanted to keep everyone from going into one of those reverent silences that ends up with people whispering to each other, as if the protagonist is dead or something. So I indulged my curiosity.

"Pierre, when you kept on about murder last night, is this what you meant?" Of course, now I was trying to include him, he shoved me out.

"No. Please, no intellectualisations. I am very unquiet, very emotional." So we did get a bit of a silence, until Sappho said, "I cannot bear that all this happened. I want to murder whoever made such pain for Orminda."

"I would like to say to you, I think in time these things pass. Even very bad things pass," said Sohan to Orminda. There is a story there, I suppose. I said something of the kind to him, and he replied in his formal way:

"You are wise. Yes. And I wish to say to you that I am very happy with the quiet way you have spoken with Orminda; just like the quiet way Chuck was speaking before with Sappho." They had had a conversation near the beginning of the morning, in which Chuck, instead of trying to curb Sappho's poutings and screechings, did a beautiful bit of straight listening. More rivalry, you would say, in my forgetting to report that.

Sappho spoke again, asking what story we were finding it so easy to find parts in. She answered herself, that it might be Hospitals. One person was patient and all the others were nurses and doctors. "Or perhaps it's just a very serious game of Mothers and Fathers," she added. My heart lightened a bit.

All through this there was an undertow of feeling as if that murder scene had happened in the next room. What I must try to get into this report are the signs of the phoenix life of this group just tapping at the egg-shell, too.

"What has just happened here is not a game. It is so powerful to me that I think perhaps it is foolish to study group behaviour. We should all go straight out and do something to stop such destruction," said Birde. For perhaps the first time, a different opinion did not sound like an attempt at annihilating the last speaker. It seemed a dignified building on what Sappho had said.

"And that destruction was also a function of group behaviour," said Pierre in a tired voice. Was he different? Or had some nasty scales dropped from my eyes? Whatever the cause, I could see him as a human, with intelligence about group behaviour. Before, I had thought he was merely clever about it.

By this time Sappho had gone to join Annie and Orminda, and was sitting on the floor in front of them, holding their legs. Out of the blue, Sappho shoved her elbow into the conversation. She spoke quietly, but the content was nothing to do with my mood, or other people's, I think. Inside me was a lump of ice that I knew would thaw into horror flowing through every vein. That was part of this moment in the group. Comforting Orminda was all, for the moment. Then Sappho said:

"I am so tired of being the responsible person! I am so tired of having insights and making the dramatisation and being the director and managing these therapeutic miracles, day after day. And instead like Pierre I see I must be the patient and the therapist and the lecturer. And the indigestion victim too, I think. That was a terrible meal last night. Perhaps this is English cooking."

To my shame, Jan, I said something absolutely crass, like, "I guess it's lunch-time." As we are serving our own food, lunch-time is totally our own affair. I added, "There's this niggle in my mind, that we shall all go so deep into the feelings round Orminda, and then maybe Sohan's story, and all the other stories we can play hospitals to..."

Birde inevitably exclaimed, "But I want that! Leave your heads and come to your senses. Perls said it." Pierre said something dark about a group illusion (Anzieu 1984) and Sohan turned to him.

"I am most anxious to learn more of these words you utter, Pierre. I seriously suggest that after lunch you explain all to us."

"Only first let's have a walk or paddle or something physical. Some change of mode," said Orminda, and thanked us simply for the morning. Some of the ice in me melted into a good flow, not horror. I have never before seen so clearly that contradiction in myself. I passionately want the group to be a shared leadership. Then I butt in and take over. That's my work area this week, or one of them.

Survival

Annie agreed with meeting a bit later, pointing out that that might mean you would be here to start the session with us.

"Perhaps this is what Pierre means when he speaks of the group illusion. Four o'clock. We meet at four o'clock," said Sappho, now twined across Chuck's legs.

"Half past three," snapped Manfred, who had been silent almost the whole morning, and whom no one had looked at, I think for at least an hour. Bad. He is sulking and we are punishing him, and I'll bet that's a scene he has got many a group to enact.

Sappho, who usually loves her own way as much as your dear little pen-pal here, said OK almost before he had finished speaking, and Pierre intoned, "Power has been given to the part of the group that experienced powerlessness."

"Do you ever speak for yourself, Pierre?" said Annie, "The Oracle is at Delphi. Omphalos Mundi. I call you Anus Monday, you are so irritating. Anus Monday, dead by Sunday." Then she looked stricken at bringing death back into the talk.

I said, "I'd like us to work out some Gestalt protocol when we meet after lunch. Responsibility language and all that stuff."

"I support that," Birde smiled at me, "And I want Pierre's contribution. And some examination of the dialogic method. And now I need us to find a way to end this group which marks our feelings. Which is more than just just shuffling off to the midday meal."

"This O of arms that Annie spoke of comes in my mind. If together, yes, like this, we make an O for Orminda." We shuffled on our knees into a circle round Orminda, with Manfred and Pierre left sitting on their chairs. Work for later. From the middle of the heap I heard Orminda's voice: "The O feels like a womb. I don't think I want to be born for a little while yet."

"Back here at four o'clock," I said.

That seems as good a place as any to stop. As I write, Orminda is sitting under a beech tree over the other side of the garden, surrounded by Sappho, Annie, Birde, Sohan, Chuck. In five minutes it will be four o'clock, and we start again. And I have not heard the taxi arriving that might be carrying you.

Jan's comment:

The preservation of the whole

What a strange and fascinating meeting. Here are nine intelligent, motivated people who have signed up to make some kind of integration of various group theories with Gestalt. So what do you do? Clam up or squabble. Like me, you have all probably lived through the same kinds of scene, and wondered who was mad. Good old Bion is my comfort at such moments. In Gestalt terms, he separated the group into the polarities of task and feeling, seeing them as two groups operant within the same population. Perhaps influenced by me, Grace suggests that you were getting into the primitive end of that feeling polarity, the Kleinian nightmare he calls the basic assumption group. Since reading Daniel Stern (1985), I think too at this stage in a new group, of the urgent process of organising data into meaning that he calls the Emergent Self.

"All learning and all creative acts begin in the domain of emergent relatedness."

I still do not know if Grace forgot that she agreed last night to the T.H. White or Merlin plan for the week, or whether Birde recorded inaccurately. Understand me, this is not about blame. It is about the weird amnesias, transpositions and substitutions that most of us, I think, make at such moments.

Accepting a blueprint from me would probably in the short term have been much easier than creating your own. And yet I see these same little psychotic glimpses in groups where I offer a blueprint. I guess the overload on that emergent self, organising principle, is going to be there whenever a number of people are going to share some of the time of their lives together. Stern talks too of affect attunement as part of the experience of intersubjectivity. Until Orminda's emotionally massive story, such attunement, identification, empathy, call it what you will, has mostly been one of what Perls called significant missing elements.

The Year Queen

Orminda's story came just when yet another fragmenting squabble was under way in a disheartened gathering.

Survival

In terms of other groups as well as this one, and in terms of the sort of role she takes in groups, there is much to be commented about this placing of her story into the wider gestalt, the whole pattern of the life of this group. She says she did something of the same in her impetuous marriage, which was sustained by a vision of national and international peace. It sounded self-neglectful, and turned out so to be.

One image that comes to the dream function of my mind, then, is of her offering herself for torture or death, for the tribe or group's sake. A quite different picture is of a wrangle of people making disguised and unsuccessful bids and counter-bids for survival, where that equates with a sense of being recognised and loved. In this, Orminda's voice might be heard as the loudest and shrillest scream, that shocked everyone into a different mode. If, on the other hand, some of people's unspoken agenda is to love and be loved, then she has certainly given a strong start to that process. The O at the end reminds me of the containing womb of the group, that can be mother to all its members.

Sometimes when I have a patient who has a persona of such sweetness and charm that she quite sets my teeth on edge, I remind myself of how often the persona is a mask for real sweetness and charm, that this person values but does not yet believe in her or himself. That same idea comes to me in groups, when there are early attempts like this to look, if not consistently be, cohesive and nurturing. Rather than discount the mask, I want to see what it is moulded on.

References

Adler A. (1929) *The Practice and Theory of Individual Psychology*. London: Kegan Paul.
Anzieu D. (1984) *The Group and the Unconscious*. Trans. B. Kilborne. London: Routledge and Kegan Paul.
Benne K. and Sheats P. (1948) Functional roles of group members, *Journal of Social Issues* **4**: 41–49.
Berne E. (1961) *Transactional Analysis in Psychotherapy*. New York: Grove Press.
Bion W. (1961) *Experiences in Groups*. London: Tavistock.
Durkin J. (Ed.) (1981) *Living Systems: Group Psychotherapy and General Systems Theory*. New York: Brunner-Mazel.

Foulkes S. H. and Anthony E. J. (1957) *Group Psychotherapy. The Psycho-Analytic Approach*. Harmondsworth: Penguin.

Freud S. (1922) *Group Psychology and the Analysis of the Ego*. Trans. J. Strachey, London: International Psycho-Analytical Press.

Frew J. Paper presented at Gestalt Journal Conference, Boston, 1992.

Goffman E. (1967) *Interaction Ritual*. New York: Doubleday.

Kelly G. (1955) *The Psychology of Personal Constructs*. New York: Norton.

Perls F. (1971). In: *Gestalt Therapy Verbatim*, New York: Bantam Books. This contribution emphasised frustration as a therapeutic method (p. 213).

Perls F., Hefferline R., Goodman P. (1951) *Gestalt Therapy. Excitement and Growth in the Human Personality*. New York: Julian Press.

Schutz W. (1966) *The Interpersonal Underworld*, Vol. 2. Palo Alto: Science and Behaviour Books, pp. 18, 25–28.

Stern D. (1985) *The Interpersonal World of the Infant*. New York: Basic Books.

Sullivan H. (1950) Tensions, interpersonal and international. In: H. Cantril (Ed.), *Tensions that Cause Wars*. Urbana: University of Illinois Press.

White T. H. (1939) *The Sword in the Stone*. London: Hart-Davis.

Wodehouse P. G. (1949) *The Mating Season* (and many other books). Harmondsworth: Penguin.

Chapter 3

Monday afternoon: Insiders and outsiders

Jan writes: People unite against a common enemy. Politicians are seen to stage-manage or even invent one, so that a troubled nation stops complaining about the economy or the government, and joins in that ultimate terrifying and exciting blood-sport, war.

In the small scale of the two groups present on the same territory at Hartley Manor, many of you seem taken quite unawares by the strength of your feelings about the in-group, the one you have apparently defended by aggression against an out-group.

You look as if you have defined the field in which you hold your awareness, as the inside of the O you made this morning, and use again this afternoon. Even I, the still-absent Jan, am part of this O. Certainly the character and history and behaviour of each member engrosses you. So the barn group are quite violently rejected as the polarity, on to which much is projected or over-projected, as emerges in the dialogue of this chapter.

Chuck's comments about the process of meeting are in line with much organisational theory (Bradford, Gibb and Benne 1964, p. 62). The sense of being taken over is quickly triggered, and leads often to florid responses. In Gestalt language, our group has maintained, or for some even momentarily achieved, a sense of its own wholeness, by closing its contact boundaries. To continue the image of a boundary, the group seems even to have made a castle wall for itself, over which ugly projections have been thrown, perhaps in some vain hope of sanitising the inner space. I remember how in Orminda's story, the murderer was outside the house.

The united front against The Others is remarkable, for a group which so far has rarely united within itself. Yet the encounter with these counsellors, and the relation to the organisers of the conference centre itself, are treated as if in parentheses, by the way. There is too much housekeeping to be done within the group, it seems, to leave people with spare attention for the rest of the world. You seem to feel yourselves as the microsphere which illustrates the way many people spend their lives. The organisational, the political, seem unpleasant and yet ignorable.

My former colleague Pat Milner uses a double entendre, possible in English, to describe Like and Not Like. Like, meaning alike, often makes or at least accompanies a first feeling of liking. Not like, meaning unalike, often leads at first to not liking. There is good sense buried in this irrationality. What seems, or is, alien, is a much stronger potential threat than what is known; so there is reason to be on guard about new scenes and new people.

Chuck's method of recording the session gives the reader scope for interpreting what is said. Without paralinguistics, which are all that is in speech besides the words, in the way of pitch, pace, pause, tone and so forth, a reader is also at a disadvantage. It is possible that at times, though, the words say it all, and the manner of speaking is a camouflage. All that is sure is that each of us will make our own contextual interpretation of what the members say.

Chuck's account

I was elected, or I sort of volunteered, to write up this session. I guess it might be the most objective just to transcribe the sound tape I ran. I got into a bit of trouble with some of the group when I let out that I was thinking of doing this.

We had met up under the beech tree at four o'clock. It was pretty warm and some of the group were there already. There was also some argy-bargy about being inside or being outside. Also, as far as I remember, about whether Sappho could smoke during the session if we were outside.

Then this nun bore down on us saying where did we want the inter-group meeting, and we all slunk off after her like dogs with our tails between our legs. It still beats me why we didn't tell her to go and stuff herself. Maybe it was the crucifix. Howsoever,

Insiders and outsiders 35

when we got back, on to the terrace round the back of the house, inside the walled garden this time, I got out the old recorder and stuck it on, and nobody said a word about it. Seems to me the group does a pretty good job of talking for themselves, anyhow. Typing this up, and clearing out the ers and ums a bit, I felt sort of impressed with what my old school teacher used to call the quality of the debate. Fancy stuff.

SAPPHO: That was an outrage! Why did we go? A whole hour when we could have been enjoying ourselves together. Nobody had told me we are forced to make politeness with these idiots.

SOHAN: It is written in the little booklet on the hall table. Also in our rooms. At the beginning and end of five-day courses, all groups in community to meet together for one hour.

ANNIE: Manfred just got up and walked after her and I followed. I agree, I didn't want to. But Grace seemed in charge. She didn't stop us.

SOHAN: I do not remember exactly, but it is written that this whole place, the Conference Centre and the Manor House, are one community.

GRACE: It's a woman who owns this place, isn't it? So we have the invisible man as our own leader, and the spectral woman causing us to face society. Weird.

CHUCK: It's all to do with the way it was set up. Sort of Desmond Morris stuff. We were sitting down, kind of submissive posture (Morris 1967) and in walks this female galleon, the bloody Armada sailing over the lawn. It was a military invasion and we were all taken prisoner. Now if we'd been in charge.... You were outrageous when we marched in there, Sappho! I loved it. "I do not like your faces. Small time people." I thought they'd lynch you.

ORMINDA: The room was so modern and hard compared with our place. I wanted them to know we had the best rooms. And I knew that would be unwise, too. Sectarian violence. I mean of course they're probably nice people really.

PIERRE: That vile personage who smiled always and spat over me as she spoke of the privilege of being part of a caring community! She smelled of fish from between the legs.

GRACE: Pierre! I could really get off on this, but we've got work of our own. That one with the moustache, though!

CHUCK: That was the Mother Superior!
BIRDE: No, she meant the rabbi, Maurice. This is wrong. It is sexism. Grace speaks not of her but of the little man like a ... what is it called? Like a gargoyle.
ANNIE: And that's not sexist? We have so much charge in hating these poor people. I suppose they are talking the same way in their group now about us.
ORMINDA: So much energy to criticise others. Perhaps we need to criticise ourselves.
GRACE: Yeah. And Jan. That's where my real hostility's directed right now. Where is the bugger?
BIRDE: This morning we spoke of reminding ourselves of Gestalt guidelines to awareness. Notice the connection of all phenomena to now. Beware of "because". Say what is going on for you; don't tell me what is going on for me. Notice images, feelings, sensations, memories, and report them for what they are. Notice the field; notice the background from which you make a figure. I have put it all on this paper, with room for more guidelines, or for objections, perhaps. Can I pin it to the bookshelves when we go inside?
ANNIE: Thank you. Let me try it. The background to that disgusting meeting just now was this delicate place in our group. We were orphan children who stopped quarrelling and took care of—I want to say of someone deeply wounded. Is that acceptable to you, Orminda?
ORMINDA: It's how I felt.
ANNIE: So now we are wonderful orphans. That is our pretence. So when these other people started to smirk and joke that our leader had not wanted to work with us, how furious I was!
BIRDE: No, it is not a pretence that we are becoming a strong group, a good group.
ANNIE: I only meant, there must be a shadow side (Jung 1928).
BIRDE: This is the folly of determinism! Jung says there is a shadow side, so you look for one. Melanie Klein (1975) says you are paranoid or depressive, so that is all you let yourselves be. Gestalt says, notice the field, the idiosyncratic field to what is figural now.
MANFRED: I quote. "*Full circle, from the tomb of the womb to the womb of the tomb, we come: an ambiguous, enigmatical incursion into a world of solid matter that is soon to melt from us, like the*

Insiders and outsiders 37

substance of a dream. And, looking back at what promised to be our own, unique, unpredictable, and dangerous adventure, all we find in the end is such a series of standard metamorphoses as as men and women have undergone in every quarter of the world, in all recorded centuries, and under every odd disguise of civilisation" (Campbell 1949, p. 12).

CHUCK: That sounds a right squelch to Birde, Manfred. What about talking for yourself, instead of reading bits of books to us? What about the old Gestalt rules, of speaking from I?

PIERRE: Have we now abandoned Jan? If we are orphans, that is what has happened.

GRACE: I'm not an orphan. I'm just looking around, putting together some of what I've learned so far. And there's Orminda's story still on my mind. I want everyone to know what you told me at lunch, Orminda. Is that all right?

ORMINDA: It's fine. It's the bit about my mother-in-law coming round earlier that evening, and me just not asking her to supper, though it was there on the table. And about all the times I wished her dead and Michael dead, and dreaded Siobhan finding out what it was not to walk properly, to have to wear a high boot.

PIERRE: The present is somehow in this story. I need to know more of the present, from everyone.

SOHAN: I hesitate, and then take the advice of Birde to tell an image. I make a fantasy of us sitting as this morning in an O round Orminda, drawing pictures of the group now. Which we can then show if we wish, and speak of.

SAPPHO: Yes, yes, yes. Anything rather than talk.

Far as I remember, Sohan gave a little pep-talk about not freezing up and thinking we'd got to be Michelangelo or someone, then he gave us these papers and some oil-pastel crayons, and fifteen minutes to do any colours or images or any old thing to do with the group. He said it clearer. But I'd switched the recorder off. I really got off on sitting on the ground doing my picture. Kind of a nursery class. The only noise was a swishing of the crayons as we all coloured away. Sohan was really put together when he got to being class teacher. He picked me up sharpish at one point when I could have got into a barney with some of the girls. It was a nice kind of a feeling, all sitting round doing the same task.

Except for our Berliner, need I say. He went off to the toilet for half the time. I said to him I didn't feel any surprise he was one of those constipated afternoon crappers.

SOHAN: If everyone has finished, let us perhaps first just arrange our pictures as we want to, without speaking. Look! It seems we make again the O, with a ring of pictures on the grass. But Orminda has gone to the side. The middle is empty.
ANNIE: The dark abyss.
GRACE: The fertile void.
BIRDE: The truth for me is that Jan is in the middle. On a throne, even. It is for him I make a fine picture. I look for him to arrive so he can see how well we do. I feel ridiculous to say it but it is true in this moment for me.
GRACE: There's a bit of that for me too. I run around the British Isles telling people that leadership is their own authority they keep projecting on to someone else. It takes one to know one. And the Jan-in-me (Weir 1982) thinks we're doing great. We're being good children by being good grown-ups.
PIERRE: What is almost overwhelming to me is the amount of material being generated here. We must make time for processing it.
SAPPHO: Look, I put my picture in the middle, then Chuck's. We are this flexible membrane to hold each other in turn. That is what I try to draw. Do you see? The group amoeba with a semi-permeable boundary. And a vacuole. That, I speak good Gestalt, represents the lacunae we keep discovering. O what a nonsense my picture is when I look again. It is an idealisation. Our semi-permeable membrane was the spines of a giant porcupine among those ugly fools at the Centre.
CHUCK: Good exercise, Sohan. I never got that sense before, of the mother-group to all the members. Just as well we can bristle up a bit when there are enemies.
SOHAN: If we wish we can each one tell also something of our pictures. Perhaps I take my turn. This little group is us setting out on a journey. We are very small. And these tigers, this is perhaps the caring community we just visited, ready to tear us to pieces. I remember, my father was agricultural worker not often in employment. When I was five years old the monsoon failed and there was no work. He led all the family, me and my

Insiders and outsiders

older sister and my two younger brothers with my mother, towards the North to find work. But no. It was a very bad journey, I must say. There, I draw flowers, to make this a fertile journey in a rich countryside. Thus was my story when my dear friend Dr Anscombe took me and my brother to England.

BIRDE: I drew aeroplanes, not very well, to show us coming from all over the world to be here. We come from everywhere! There is a song: The whole world, in my hand; I've got the whole world in my hand.

CHUCK: Funny bloody world here, with no China, no Far East at all beyond India; no South America; no Africa except at a few removes. Let's not get carried away.

BIRDE: I feel as if hit. I imagine you express that you like Sappho and that you despise me. But you disguise in reasons what you feel.

SOHAN: Perhaps for now we go on with what Sappho started, we tell the pictures. Later we discuss.

CHUCK: Point taken. Sorry.

BIRDE: Without censoring, I heard a robin, and drew also a nest with many birds. O, I had not seen! There are nine! In Scandinavia I feel often that I am far from people who understand me. To be here is somehow to come back to the nest. I think perhaps for Manfred it is the same.

MANFRED: I have nothing to say about my picture. I'm not sure why I joined in the exercise at all. I'm not interested in drawing.

ANNIE: I notice how intensely embarrassed I feel. The impulse is just to smile and pretend that it's OK for you not to say anything personal. But I'm not going to muzzle myself. You've drawn something very small, Manfred, in about ten seconds. I can't make it out, right up in one corner. I partly want to shout at you. And I really admired that you walked out of that blasted community meeting after about three minutes. I wish we'd followed you that time too.

MANFRED: I am making some private experiments around exclusion.

SAPPHO: O, congratulations! And what am I supposed to do with that? Maybe I make some experiments at you, in ostracism. This is not a laboratory! I am real! Orminda was real this morning!

MANFRED: That is your problem, not mine. I think it is written so in your so-called Gestalt prayer.

GRACE: You're a puzzle to me, Manfred. Last night you came on strong, showed us some family therapy. What happened? What changed? It's like you left us.

CHUCK: Leave him be. I'll display my art work. These are supposed to be pigs. No offence. I was thinking of the fairy story. We've all got these weird lumps of building material, see, and we're kind of trying to make one house out of them. And then over here there's the old wolf. I don't know if it's Jan or the Caring Community we behaved so badly in, or what. But the old wolf sure is huffing and puffing at us; and we sure don't know if our little house will hold together.

ANNIE: There's some connection with mine there. I've got us sitting in a room with artificial light. Sort of false clarity. And we cast these big dark shadows that make this writhing shape underneath us. And under that, hidden by the shadows, is some archetypal anchor that binds us together. I just drew, I didn't think too much at the time.

ORMINDA: I've put myself in the middle. I've been outside everything for all these months. But now I'm here and I've got all this yellow light streaming in on me from everyone, and streaming out of me.

SAPPHO: Catharsis.

GRACE: And I can feel that too. But what I drew... Like Annie, I'm going to say it, but it would be easier to avoid. Look, I've got us with the shot father and the shot baby. They're not even in coffins yet for me. There's that reality, and all our different fears about hate and envy and death and pairing and violence to make into some sort of compost. Or what Chuck calls building material, yes, a better image. That's why I put all these spades at the side. A lot of digging to do.

MANFRED: I am sure we all agree that Grace once again wins the group competition for the best contribution.

GRACE: Ouch. That hurt. I know I am competitive.

SOHAN: I do assure you that this is a co-operation, not at all a competitive exercise.

MANFRED: How cosy.

SAPPHO: Grace says something that is not at all cosy. So much stirs inside me at this picture. At all the pictures. They are like those transparencies for teaching aids—one goes on top of another and you understand more. I want your transparency,

Insiders and outsiders

Manfred. O, you are so frustrating when you sit thus and stay silent!
ANNIE: It is easy for you to be transparent, Sappho. I imagine you as the pretty child, the secure adored one in your family. For some of us being seen, being transparent...
PIERRE: Birde says speak from the first person.
ANNIE: For me to be seen too much feels almost like being eaten up. The feeling is there and I work to overcome it; but I want to say it too.
GRACE: Sohan, thank you very much for your exercise. You helped me know more.
SOHAN: One day perhaps we do another.
SAPPHO: Tonight! Let's do another tonight. Or else dance. Who has some tapes?
BIRDE: Before tonight there is eating. Why do we not do as these other groups on low budget in the Centre, and cook for ourselves? I spoke with this Mrs Peters who makes the tough spaghetti and crunching beans. She only comes because the real helper is on holiday, and the substitute has a broken leg. She would be very happy only to do shopping for us, and prepare vegetables and salad.
SAPPHO: But I wanted to leave all the real world behind. Cooking! Pooh!
CHUCK: Anything to reduce the fart level. I came down those stairs jet-propelled after lunch. I'll do us an Aussie barbie one night if you like.
SOHAN: I would be happy to offer some Indian dish not too spicy for Western taste on another occasion.
GRACE: Manfred, if people agree, would you organise a rota for cooking?
MANFRED: Of course. Such a thing is easily done. On Tuesday we shall need for the breakfast meal one person or two persons, who will report...
GRACE: If you'd just do it and put a list or tell people, outside group time.
BIRDE: I have been in so many training groups where to smoke or not to smoke, to have ten or twenty minutes for coffee, to start at two o'clock or five past or half past, has been such intense discussion. We're fast deciders.
PIERRE: Les ennuis couvrent l'ennui.

GRACE: O my God. Now he speaks in foreign tongues too. Pierre, you're definitely on parade after supper. Whether Jan marches in or not.

ANNIE: Grace is the perfect mother of this group. Pierre is the stern father. Sohan and Orminda are our lovely children. Chuck is the exciting cousin come to visit. Sappho is the naughty girl from next door. Birde and I are two aunts, not quite accepted as belonging by others, though we feel ourselves part of the family.

SAPPHO: Yes, Aunty.

MANFRED: Orne says, *"Persons make meaning and order even in the absence of meaning and order".*

PIERRE: Or perhaps, in the penumbra of many meanings, many levels of meaning and order, Annie expresses one that is disturbing to you.

BIRDE: It is definitely time for stern father to tell us the meaning of life.

SAPPHO: Some time I wish private conversation with Birde. I reject your antagonism to me.

PIERRE: Perhaps you speak for more of the group than yourself. Perhaps antagonism is rejected here.

GRACE: After supper! And let's put our pictures up, so Jan can see some of our hopes and fears and fantasies.

Jan's comment

As in the morning, the shape of the session is a move away from perturbations at the beginning. Sohan has reminded people that there will be another inter-group meeting before the end of the week. Chuck has suggested that such a meeting could be handled more proactively. But there the topic has died, maybe less from natural causes, like living its full life to the end, but rather, in mysterious circumstances. A collective forgetting or neglect occurs.

We do not know if the summer's day, the menace of this outgroup, Orminda's plight, or what all else are the influences in the field. What does show is a move in the group to more cohesion for more of the time. Sohan comments how people place their pictures in a circle when they have finished. The image is elaborated: the group as container for the members in turn. Another

Insiders and outsiders

way to express this is as I did when that O first occurred: a group which is womb or mother to each member. The group is then an idealised retreat. This aspect shows perhaps in the vilification of the outsider group. It may also be in Birde's picture of a nest full of nine birds. Only young dependent birds inhabit nests.

As in all groups, I imagine a hierarchy of needs (Goldstein 1939). If so, the present need seems to be nest-building rather than moving into the macrosphere (Erickson 1951).

Chuck's picture of pigs and building material is still childish, but it is about effort, construction, intention. It connects to the conversation near the end, about taking over the cooking, and offering each other national dishes. Eating is a central theme of Gestalt theory (Perls 1947). Taking over the kitchen sounds a bit like moving on from being spoon-fed. Feeding is nurturing, mothering, in this context, so self-catering is perhaps a mature experiment in creating the mother-group.

Birde spells out some Gestalt guidelines, and this too looks like the building of a group methodology. It is noticeable, though, that there is no comment on what she says. In the eating analogy, there is no chewing, no assimilating. Nor is there rejection, at least overtly. So there may be the swallowing whole of introjection.

A bit of chewing that is attempted is when Manfred is confronted for refusing to talk about his picture. Grace, who makes a number of group-management interventions, does not swallow his devaluing. Then later, with deftness, she invites him to organise a rota. If this is meant to include him in the O, it succeeds, at least for him. But Annie rejects him clearly, by simply omitting him when she draws a word-picture of the group as a family (Yalom 1985).

Pierre is teased rather than berated in this session. And he is warmly invited or bullied to comment on the evening meeting. He is apparently in the club, and behaves that way himself. Manfred is left to carry the outsider role, and co-operates disastrously, with his talk of private experiments in exclusion.

The image of orphans suggests that, for the moment at least, I am deemed dead for some of you. Whether this is to do with resignation or wish-fulfilment is not clear. The corollary is that the children are getting on with their own lives. In all the complexity of this task, it looks as if many of you have settled on one simplification. What is bad is outside the group. At moments it is clear that Manfred is classified thus, and treated accordingly.

Organism shaped by field

Within the group, storming, norming and performing have to some extent succeeded each other. Having the counsellor group brought to awareness as part of the field has probably been an influence in group formation. The same hostile and competitive feelings that showed between members within the Manor group, now appear in more caricature ways in relation to the outgroup. A simple polarity is invented, between good and bad. A corollary is implicit: the bad is to be ignored.

It could be said that Manfred represents whatever is styled the bad within each person, and becomes part of a group dramatisation of a personal intrapsychic process. It could as well be argued that in the field of five days, without the advantage of an informed leader, and with the mind-bending task of reconciling or at least comparing several theories of group process with Gestalt, it would be a waste of time to cope with an unco-operative group member; the survival of the majority is more important. Both explanations have relevance.

Many therapy and training groups concentrate, rightly, on the rich material within the group boundary. Imports and exports from the group happen via every member, without necessarily being figural. Now all of you are faced as-a-group with how to create and use a contact boundary. Osmotic membrane and porcupine spines are talked of. In other words, there is not a hint of confluence with the outgroup, who sound as if they have much in common with all of you.

In the field of the group, Manfred will be shaped by the attitudes and behaviour of the other members towards him, as well as vice versa. In the field of the conference centre, you are similarly being influenced by what is happening between you and the counselling group. The same hopes and suspicions that are being dealt with between the members of our group, are floridly, caricaturedly possible between the larger entities of the two groups. Being a group member *in the field which includes the out-group* looks notably different from self-perception *as a member within the group*. Suddenly, and maybe briefly, you seem as a group to have a lot in common with a walnut, with a pretty hard shell to the outside.

References

Bradford L., Gibb J. and Benne K. (1964) *T-Group Theory and Laboratory Method*. New York: John Wiley.

Campbell A. (1949) *The Hero with a Thousand Faces*. Princeton, NJ., Princeton University Press.

Erickson E. (1951) *Childhood and Society*. London: Imago.
>   Erickson describes three realities. These are, first, the autosphere of infancy, where only the body is real, then the microsphere of play and transference, and last the macrosphere, the outer zone of agreed reality. These have overlap with Perls' notion of inner, middle and outer zones.

Fairbairn M. (1954) *The Object Relations Theory of Personality*. New York: Basic Books.

Goldstein K. (1939) *The Organism*. New York: American Book Co.
>   Goldstein, who had contact with Perls and Goodman, coined the term self-actualisation, some time before Abraham Maslow made it well known.

Jung C. (1928) *Contributions to Analytical Psychology*. London: Kegan Paul, Trench, Trubner, pp. 256–258.

Klein M. (1975) *Envy and Gratitude and Other Works 1946–1963*. New York: Julian Press.

Morris D. (1967) *The Naked Ape*. London: Jonathan Cape.

Perls F. (1947) *Ego, Hunger and Aggression*. London: Allen and Unwin.

Perls F., Hefferline R. and Goodman P. (1951) *Gestalt Therapy*. New York: Dell.

Stern D. (1985) *The Interpersonal World of the Infant*. New York: Basic Books.

Weir J. (1982) Percept language. In: G. Houston (Ed.), *The Red Book of Gestalt*. London: Rochester Foundation, pp. 62–66.

Yalom I. (1985) *The Theory and Practice of Group Psychotherapy*. New York: Basic Books, p. 392.

Chapter 4

Monday evening: Thurber's war

Jan writes: I notice the amount of dread with which I picked up this fourth account of a session at which I was still not present. Perls often spoke of the schizophrenic levels of the mind. I would say I have been in and out of the paranoid levels of mine. I guess it is to do with a right-minded assessment that if nine of you gang up on me physically, I have not much of a hope of survival. Surely that is what underlies the fear of the group that so many people experience, before they have their place a little secure.

Once more I feel the double bind of having only words to describe what is before and under and alongside words. I can make such glittering facile patterns of words, and so deceive myself with them. And I feel awe at the subtlety, the nuance of meaning they allow to be communicated. I always had trouble with the idea of the Word being made Flesh (Gospel according to St. John). To my mind, trouble started when the Flesh was made Word. I see why these thoughts come to me as I read Pierre's report. Much of it is about fragmenting, sub-grouping, schism, that might be more clearly perceived by movement than description.

Pierre's account

As I listen to this tape I see that I make many omissions of interpretation. I am the circus performer attempting to ride two horses, Gestalt and psychoanalysis. Strong sexual motivations are disguised in my so-called co-operative lapses into Gestalt mode, I think. If only I had some observers with whom to discuss my own pathology in this process (Anzieu 1984).

Thurber's war

Certainly the writing up is my own leadership bid formalised. I experience what Marx and Engels (1847) call the power of the secretariat.

I resist a strong temptation to justify the completely idiotic role I take in much of this session. First I play helpful group member. At some moments I interpret individuals, argue, impose myself, and so take many conflicting roles without explanation. It is as if I try to comment on the Atlantic Ocean while sitting on a minuscule raft on it in the middle of a tornado. Too much emotion is present for me to think coolly. Too much material presents too quickly. Tomorrow I shall refuse an evening session, I think. My view is reinforced that without observers and some supervisory conversation after the meeting, it is impossible to make much intelligent interpretation (Foulkes and Anthony 1957).

My observation in this group is no doubt very biassed. My abstinence is in question. I do not disclose all. So I am a bad analytic group leader. Perhaps this overwhelmed subjectivity is seen as authentic Gestalt leadership.

From this storm-tossed position I think I discern a fight between me and Chuck, expressed as differences of philosophy. And I accept also what I had not seen at the time, a grouping of the sexes against each other. Even the first words of the transcript make this clear; but I ignored all.

ANNIE: Look. The men are all huddling together tonight.
SAPPHO: I make a metamorphosis. Move your chair, Pierre. I sit among you.
PIERRE: I have no wish to move my chair.
SOHAN: Here is a space I make, Sappho.
BIRDE: Where's Manfred? We've waited nearly ten minutes. I want to start. All the rest of us can get here on time.
SAPPHO: He re-builds the Berlin Wall from academic books. Or makes more permutations of his list. I hate this list! Gestalt is of spontaneity. Grace, it was you who gave him this little job. So patronising. So catastrophic. The gruppenfuehrer is created to oppress us with his presence and with his absence.
BIRDE: I feel oppressed by you, Sappho. It made me uncomfortable that you approached me at lunch and requested with me a private conversation. Then when I came to you at supper you waved your hand and said "Later, later".

SAPPHO: I was speaking with Pierre and Chuck.
BIRDE: Precisely.

Several minutes passed.

ORMINDA: What is the matter with us tonight? We're so heavy. The silences go on so long.
GRACE: I'm listening for the phone in case Jan suddenly rings. And I'm not going to answer it, by the way. Consider that buck passed.
ANNIE: And that open door really disturbs me. I want us enclosed. Manfred and Jan are both the other side of it somewhere. In, or out, please. I don't want a swinging door.
CHUCK: I guess we all have our different reasons for being slow. I'm waiting for Pierre to do his bit. Shit or get off the pot. Wasn't that one of Perls' little mottoes?
PIERRE: Perhaps the struggle for the group is to do with the swinging door.
GRACE: You're all good at English; but you have some funny phrases. And I slow down my speech for you. But with you, Pierre, it's not just the accent. You look as if you're concentrating furiously, then you say stuff like that. I believe you mean something. Please. Allow for what I guess you would call my resistance. I think it's just a language deficiency. Plato (*Thaeatetus*) said a beautiful bit about language not reflecting the flux, the process. *The verb "to be" should be deleted from all contexts... We should instead adapt our speech to the way things are, and describe them as undergoing generation, production, destruction and alteration ... speech which suggests stability is easily refuted* (p. 40). So speak to me in Gestalt, please. "I". The concrete example. The owned fantasy.
PIERRE: "Funny phrases," you said. "Uncomfortable," Birde said earlier. I have the impression that you Gestaltists inhibit, to avoid conflict. Conflict, hostility, anger, hate, envy, spite: all these are outside the group, outside the door some people wish closed. Then in here perhaps we are the good group who takes care of the wounded. I have this wish in me also, yes. I remember my indignation at this big group we were forced to go to. I made it so bad, to contain all the badness. I see this truth and I distrust my affect, my feelings.

SOHAN: O excuse me, that I interrupt what is so interesting. But I think I am seeing Manfred on the path. Manfred! O.
CHUCK: What did he say? I couldn't hear.
SOHAN: He said. He goes to pub with other group.
GRACE: What have we done that drives him out? I nearly said, that drives him to the arms of another woman?
CHUCK: Straight. I am not going to spend the evening talking about that bastard. How come you look so cut up about him, Sohan?
PIERRE: Sohan has internalised the group.
BIRDE: Say I, say I. You do not know what Sohan has done.
PIERRE: He registers the loss of male energy to what is already a threatened group. So the question arises, what sin has been committed here, that we are punished in this way?
GRACE: I just said that, in different words. Didn't you hear me?
CHUCK: Jesus, Pierre! It's just a simple power-struggle. That bastard wants to run this group, and you stop him. That's as clear as the nose on your smug face. Just don't give me this psychoanalytic crap about sin and schism. You changed your whole image around, halfway through what you were saying. First we're keeping sin out, then we're guilty anyway. Bloody Sunday School without the hymns. I like Sappho's idea of a song and a dance. Can't we get up and boogie a little?
PIERRE: In this way the illusion of goodness can be preserved. We shall perhaps forget that women can be so full of hate that they kill.
CHUCK: Since the moment you walked in here you've been dead keen. O, that's weird. Thank you, Sigmund. You've been on the trail of thanatos, boy.
SOHAN: Excuse me, I do not know this word.
CHUCK: It's a crap idea from Freud, of a death instinct. Mind you, I can kind of get in touch with it when I look at Pierre.
PIERRE: If you have to fight me so vigorously, perhaps I represent an idea that you resist.
CHUCK: I resist the idea that the moon's made of green cheese. I resist stark idiocy.
PIERRE: You work as a psychiatrist. Is this a symbol of resisting your own madness, of seeking always to cure or contain the psychotic?

Now came a silence full of turmoil.

CHUCK: Where did we get to? I can't remember what was happening before we all drifted into this kind of trance. Is that the phone? Well go, somebody! Look, it's the phone. Won't someone answer it? OK, OK. I'll be the sacrificial lamb.

We waited without speaking till he came back.

CHUCK: I get the impression that this has not been a scintillating gathering in my brief absence. In fact I would say there are very few vital signs.
SAPPHO: Was it Jan?
CHUCK: Yup. Now in Salonika. I told him he should have gone to Thessaloniki.
SAPPHO: It is the same place.
CHUCK: What? Anyway, the Salonika airport's out in sympathetic strike action. I felt sorry for the bugger. I told him we were doing fine, and to make it when he could. That kind of stuff.
PIERRE: How many men have to go before we stop being a group?
BIRDE: O, I am angry. Five women sit here and you take no notice of us. I am in many wonderful groups that are of all women, or women with only one or two men. But I hear you saying that if men go, the group is no more.
ANNIE: A long while back, Grace said something, about what we had done to make Manfred go. The men went straight on talking, then Pierre said what she had said, as if it was a new thought.
BIRDE: Yes. She said it much more to the point than Pierre did, I think.
GRACE: Either the women have the floor, or the men do. I imagine us in two camps. You know what I heard myself singing as I walked in here? "You've read in the Bible, or you've been told, The battle of the sexes ten thousand years old." That didn't come from nowhere, O no.
SOHAN: Tonight I learn so much, with such alarms, such clutching in my stomach.
ORMINDA: Till you spoke, Sohan, I was just so angry at this male conversation. You looked at each other, Pierre and Chuck mostly, and just cued each other to speak, so there was never a gap or an invitation to the women. Oo! Men!

GRACE: Manfred suggested a half past three meeting for this afternoon. And Birde agreed. We all did. I know I was placating Manfred. He seemed so hurtable and difficult.

BIRDE: Please speak of you, not of someone absent.

GRACE: Point taken. Then right at the end I said something like, "See you all at four o'clock". And that is in fact when we met. Quite unawarely, I took away his victory, and substituted a petty one of my own. (Perls, Hefferline and Goodman 1951). When I say that, I remember Pierre's words. In a way I was like Orminda's mother-in-law. I laid in wait and shot him.

ORMINDA: Before that, I displaced him in the group to sit near Sohan.

GRACE: And I don't remember anyone saying anything appreciative about his readings and stuff.

ORMINDA: You looked right at me as you spoke. It's very good to meet your eyes. I want to embrace you. Thank you. That is very good. Thank you, Buber (1970). And now I want Pierre to join the hug.

PIERRE: Excuse me. I think still of what you say of Manfred. It is as if you describe the Last Supper in John's Gospel. The disciples acted as such idiots! As you did. So stupid! Judas Iscariot carried their bad feelings, which as holy men they denied in themselves. So when Christ said that one of them would betray him, they simply made a concourse of which of them was the most lovable. Then one asks for a sign of who the betrayer was. Christ spelled it out. "I give a sop to the betrayer." He gives a sop to Judas and tells him to do what he has to do. Still the disciples act dumb. They think Jesus is telling him to do the shopping! No, you do not remember this! Look it up in the Bible. But you are more honest than the twelve. You admit your complicity in Manfred's defection. That is already progress. But this hug has the smell of seduction. It would be what I think you call bad faith (Sartre 1943) for me to join you.

BIRDE: Look at your hand, Pierre. When you said no, you stretched it towards Orminda. Words can lie. Bodies are more in good faith, I think.

CHUCK: If you'd accept substitutes, Orminda, I guess Sohan or I...?

SAPPHO: Can't we dance? Grace started singing before. Let's get up. I can see one of those group hugs imminent. Intolerable.

ORMINDA: This morning I felt very small, and I wanted the group round me as a kind of faceless comfort. Now I feel more grown-up. I see you all separately. I'd hate to have a group hug, too.

GRACE: I'm noticing all this war between the sexes inside me. In my sort of ordinary reasoning reasonable brain I'd say that I have only good feelings to Chuck and Sohan. To Manfred, there's a lot of irritation; there's also a therapist feeling, an alarm light that he's at risk here. To Pierre I have the strongest feelings. Huge resistance at moments. Then I feel an excitement, little cold lines running down my arms, as I notice how the images I use overlap with these observations you make. And I respect that you make efforts to take a Gestalt perspective, Pierre. Sometimes.

SAPPHO: I have no problem with men.

BIRDE: Perhaps it is this makes problems for me. You sit close to them and touch them and look often in their faces.

ANNIE: What you said of the swinging door was very useful to me, Pierre. In my language, we are still in the paranoid schizoid position, and struggling against moving to the depressive (Klein 1957).

No one spoke for a time.

BIRDE: Again the trance! (Rossi 1986) I feel first stubborn that you use these dark and gloomy words, Annie. Then I am stuck, feeling tender towards Orminda still, as in many silences, but fearing always to change the subject.

SOHAN: And what happens if you change the subject?

BIRDE: I shall be the bad person and you will not love me.

GRACE: There is so much to take in. I know how to run groups so people feel safe, and get insights, and gain depth. I know how to be a good member in such groups. And now I have the chance to move outside my competence. Instead of just knowing about, I can subject myself to this way of looking at what I suppose Annie and Pierre call unconscious forces. The amount of scare I feel is strange. The dark abyss, Annie said.

ORMINDA: I think I'm feeling something the same. I've been troubled at times, at having done something quite violent to the group by telling what I told this morning.

Thurber's war

BIRDE: You gave opportunity for us to show tenderness. This is a gift you gave us.

ORMINDA: And was it a blackmail too? How can anyone be nasty to me when I have suffered such a tragedy? Or, worse. Did I throw this story of hate at you, so we are all paranoid now, as Annie perhaps says? I don't quite follow her theory. I mean, was I saying a double bind message (Bateson 1972), that I demand peace, but that I know there is hate and murder and betrayal and callousness really?

GRACE: What I notice now is a letting go of tension in my neck and shoulders. I associate that partly to what you are saying, Orminda, and partly to a change between the men and women. For me the battle of the sexes is over. Is it true for others? More is out in the open.

PIERRE: Orminda makes a fearless interpretation. She sees herself as not just this person to whom an almost intolerable tragedy has occurred. She also uses that part of her life here, for present purposes, which could be maladaptive, or what you call growthful. Or both.

SAPPHO: Just for me, Pierre! Teach us to make interpretations. I had this English boy-friend, what did he say? Don't knock it till you've tried it.

GRACE: It's almost like sinking back in my head, so my thoughts slow or go, and images come up.

PIERRE: This is an excellent advice. Allow metaphor to have live meaning. Notice puns, paradoxes, curious affect.

SOHAN: Affect, please?

PIERRE: Feelings. Let in the poetic mode, the inconsequences, the taboo. And do not censor. So we have the rule to disclose...

GRACE: Like the Gestalt, "Be as open as you can". And there's a bit in Perls, Hefferline and Goodman (1951, p. 326) that I remember: *The poet...richly develops the symbols with a lively use of his senses, projecting* himself...*rather than alienating.*

PIERRE: ...and the rule of abstinence. We perhaps speak of strange things. We do not do them.

GRACE: Like the usual group rule of no violence.

PIERRE: So, I step back as Grace says to this mental position of not being caught in primary processes. What is going on between us in the group, that she makes a false likeness between analysis and Gestalt?

CHUCK: A kind of a power struggle.

ANNIE: Back to the swinging door. If Gestalt and psychoanalysis are comprehensible and mostly the same, then this group is all good, is the good mother of good children. Dissension and bad feeling are outside.

GRACE: Yes. But. I see I'm yes-butting. So I am. We have plenty of dissension here, and own it.

ORMINDA: And ever and anon I flit to this fantasy that everything will be all right here. More than that. That somehow I shall be altogether healed here.

SOHAN: Very much I hope that this will be so. And yet I am knowing we are somewhat helpless before so great a loss.

ANNIE: I've kept having moments of dread. I tell myself it's to do with Jan not arriving. And Manfred being so—well, he is, difficult. Grace said that strange, that disturbing thing, of seeing a glimpse of that mother-in-law in her. That would have been difficult for me to admit. But now you've done it, Grace, I let myself see how I can be this little Siobhan who will never walk properly, and who does not even realise that. I'm sorry I'm crying. Take no notice.

SAPPHO: You can walk! You can walk! You have two good legs.

BIRDE: It is a metaphor.

SAPPHO: Of course it is a metaphor. I know that. I wish she uses a different one. With this metaphor she makes her life bad. It is an enchantment she puts on herself (Bettelheim 1976).

GRACE: Last night Birde spoke of Merlin. I do feel as if I am working to keep some spells at bay. And I am trying to cast my own, I suppose.

BIRDE: This is a very fine group. It is a privilege to be part of it.

PIERRE: Birde pronounces the enchantment that she wishes for, and which she repeats already many times. Perhaps she fears her spell is not strong enough to keep reality aux abois—at bay.

SAPPHO: You know what I think? I think Jan makes an experiment on us. He writes of the autonomous group. By his absence he tries if we can be one. Perhaps he really does watch from that great fireplace, or behind a screen.

BIRDE: While I think he does such things, I am not autonomous. I am still dependent on him, I think. At some moments this group is in life like a great panther leaping through the jungle. Then I see us as once more some grubs in a cheese, fat and

Thurber's war

even blinded by so much food around us, and not organised. It is too grown-up, it is too soon to be so leaderless.

PIERRE: I have many feelings in regard to leadership. I am in rivalry with you, Grace. I indulge in inward sneering. Not good. Also, this image of the grubs in the cheese has great power for me.

ANNIE: The great panther has leapt for me at times when you have taken Grace's hand instead of turning away from her.

PIERRE: This I accept. I dread the phallic mother.

GRACE: Who's she? I guess I'd dread her if I saw her coming down the street. With her bosom and her codpiece.

ORMINDA: There's quite a desperate sound in our laughter.

CHUCK: It's a desperate bloody image. You know, we could send ourselves crazy here, sitting exchanging these mad dreams.

ORMINDA: I remember being in a group in the States, and an American Indian getting us to bring our dreams each morning and tell them. Rank speaks of the idea the Iroquois have, that waking life is the dream, and dreams the reality.

PIERRE: The group itself is a dream.

BIRDE: Let's do that tomorrow. Start by telling our dreams.

The tape machine is most helpful to reveal the moments when we colluded to pass into a trance. I see these moments almost as an electrical short, a response to overload of threat, perfectly sustained by all members. There were more than the long ones I have noted. These came, first, when Sappho appeared to have cornered the male sexual energy; next, at my suggestion that the group was resisting its own madness; then, when Chuck left the group, to speak to yet another missing male. It is to be noted also that he described himself in doing so as a sacrificial lamb. In these pauses perhaps we have clues to all the work that needs to be done in this group.

At first the idea is discussed that badness is exterior to the group. Then Manfred walks by, exterior to the group, rejecting us, defecting to the enemy. Then comes the female attempt to enfold him, even in his absence, to forgive him and draw him back into membership. I have seldom had such a strong sense of the honest work-group recovering from an unconscious collusion to destroy, to scapegoat, one member. How we treat him now is of great interest to me.

The talk with Chuck before this I enjoyed. I note that I had omitted to mention it, and note too that there are many forces resisting the enjoyment of the homosexual sub-group (Freud 1912) and the rejection of the other sex. I and Chuck for a moment were members of the English Gentleman's Club in the West End, until the guilt-inducing feminist hordes reproached us.

The image of irresistible sirens comes to me. But there is no one to bind me to the mast.

There is great good will in this group to learn the interpretative mode. I do not know if the true work-group emerges, however. It is possible that tokens of collaboration are introduced, as spells to ward off disintegration and schism.

Tomorrow I circulate these notes for comment by other members. For Jan, I think not. As a professional Gestaltist, I suppose his resistance to my assumptions and methods.

Jan's comment

The Thurber war between the sexes reminds me of Bennis and Shepard (1956) who describe phases of group life with great exactitude. In their terms, our group is at the stage of forming two warring sub-groups. In Frew's (1986) schema of three phases of group life, you sure look as if you are in the middle one, *conflict*, rather than *orientation*, or the *cohesion* he names as his third phase. Again, in Bion's language, fight and flight are still discernible modes. As some of you probably know, George Bach (1954) made a seven-phase description of group life. Well, I never was in a group that held to his or anyone else's schema, unless I shoved it a little. Yet every one of these theories has helped me make sense of certain groups at certain times. Here in this report, you are in too rich an experience for me to reduce to a short descriptive phrase.

That the gender wrangle has started is in Gestalt an indication that people are ready to let it start. What was before experienced as moments of pique by individuals is now an aware sub-grouping. It has come out of the dark of the half-aware, into awareness. This schism has been foreshadowed at earlier moments. The Gestalt slogan, separate to integrate, makes a good deal of sense here. The attraction between the sexes, at sexual level, seems likely to be considerable among relatively young, vigorous, apparently heterosexual, in some ways like-minded people who are living in the same building and far from home. A drawing back to look at each other, and the making of solidarity within the same-sex group, looks a pretty good idea to the observer. I certainly go along with Bach's idea that our group is probably at the high-awareness-of-ingroup stage now.

Pierre's Last Supper story is a whole-group view of a betrayal for which one person can be scapegoated. It counteracts the less clearly expressed wish to purify the group by getting rid of the deviant member. I notice that he wants to keep these notes away from me. Both attitudes make the whole-group figural, either by including or excluding.

As I read, the image came to my awareness of a walnut. I saw the group as this lobed and wrinkled entity, almost two cerebral hemispheres, one female and one male. The different members seemed like lobes, surface protruberances from the matrix. And round you was a pretty complete shell. That is curious, as you do not act united too much of the time. But I sure feel on the outside.

Another polarity is personified between Pierre, who represents a focus on pathology and id-process, and Grace, who represents the Gestalt focus on excitement and growth, and ego-processes, those within awareness.

Not content with an ingroup and outgroup, with Manfred as bad guy to the rest as OK, the group I see as a walnut just now is stuffed with conflicting polarities. Ego and id. Men and women. Leader and group. Feeling and task.

Reality-testing and the creation of myths seem to be galloping together at moments in this process. So there is another polarity, along with Pierre's hinted one of strong attraction and its polarity, fear.

Separation is a stage towards new integration. Rather than acknowledge physis, the unified life energy that might be in all action, you are intent on splitting, and then scrapping. What for?

Maybe your fighting shows that you matter enough to each other to get upset about. Development of the group and the people in it depends on whether enough of you become a force for contact, integration and change. Aggression and destructuring are the Gestalt description of the next growthful possibilities. *Aggression* in Gestalt language is simply, in its root Latin sense, vigorous outward-directed activity. Destruction, as Perls uses the word here, means destructuring, as in winnowing: *The process of mutual destruction is probably the chief proving ground of profound compatibility* (Perls, Hefferline and Goodman 1951, p. 342)

References

Anzieu D. (1984) *The Group and the Unconscious*. Trans. Kilborne B. London: Routledge and Kegan Paul.
Bach G. (1954) *Intensive Group Psychotherapy*. New York: Ronalds Press.
Bateson G. (1972) The logical categories of information and learning. In: *Steps to an Ecology of Mind*. New York: Ballantyne Books.
Bennis W. and Shepard H. (1956). In: G. Gibbard, J. Hartman and R. Mann (Eds), *Analysis of Groups*. San Francisco: Jossey Bass, 1974.
Bettelheim B. (1976) *The uses of Enchantment*. London: Thames and Hudson.
Buber M. (1970) *I and Thou*. New York: Scriveners.
Foulkes S. and Anthony E. (1957) *Group Psychotherapy—The Psycho-Analytic Approach*. Harmondsworth: Penguin.
   These innovative practitioners saw immense value in free-floating group discussion, and assert that we do not know the value of interpretation. Perls went further, and proscribed interpretation, except perhaps by the protagonist.
Freud S. (1912) *Totem and Taboo*. Standard edition, Vol. 13, London: Hogarth Press, 1955.
Frew J. (1986) The functions and patterns of occurrences of individual contact styles during the developmental phases of the gestalt group. *Gestalt Journal* **9**: 55–70.
Gospel according to St. John, Ch. 13, 23–29.
Klein M. (1957) *Envy and Gratitude*. London: Tavistock.
Marx K. and Engels F. (1847) *Manifest der Kommunistischen*. London.
Perls F., Hefferline R. and Goodman P. (1951) *Gestalt Therapy*, Vol. 2, Ch.9. New York: Julian Press.
Plato, *Theaetetus*, Trans. R. Waterfield. Harmondsworth: Penguin, 1987.
Rossi E. (1986) *The Psychobiology of Mind-Body Healing*. New York: W.W. Norton.
Sartre J.-P. (1943) *L'Etre et le Neant*. Paris: Gallimard.

Chapter 5

Tuesday morning: The dream of leadership

Jan writes: What promise and what threat you all must have represented to each other, maybe the more so with me still absent. It must be rare to work alongside so many people competent at the edge of your own field. In this group where the roles are not clear or pre-ordained, one unstated and emotionally urgent task, I guess, is for all of you to get recognition *as professionals*. John Frew would call this the Differentiation stage of the group, Schutz the Control phase. Both see competition as a big task at such a time.

Looking now at Sappho's account of this session, I have enough distance to see the theme of leadership style. But Sappho is within the group, experiencing the stimulus of rivalry. In a letter she wrote me lately, she agreed that you as followers were less willing to follow, than she as leader was to lead. The abrupt change to a transcript at a certain point in the report suggests the extent to which she and the rest of you were out of line.

The struggle is a significant one, between someone whose personality warms to clear goal-setting and Apollonic leadership (Handy 1991), and the tendency among some of the group towards the pure examination of the moment. She may see this as a diffuse and Dionysiac indulgence.

Having the answers is useful in a leader, where saving time or effort are important. As an enemy tank bears down on the platoon, it is not the moment for democratic consultation. But when Sappho thinks she knows Chuck has suffered sexual abuse, she gives him no psychic space. The illusion is that time and effort are saved. Reality is that more will be needed in the long run, to deal with the intrusion, and re-establish rapport. I labour the point, and I hope Sappho will forgive me. What she shows is a style that it is all too easy for managers, bosses and therapists to use. The more competent they become, often the greater the temptation to provide rather than elicit.

Leadership is partly to do with imposing. Unless there is also synergy between leader and led for enough of the time, there is always trouble. Organising the field in this way, I notice that almost the first overt task undertaken this morning is the telling of dreams, which Orminda proposed, and Birde warmly seconded last night. Birde attempts to shape the dream-telling, but is opposed by Sappho. From the start, there is clear imposition in Sappho's style.

Her own assessment of where she acknowledges authority, recognised leadership in the group at the moment, may show in the first lines of her writing.

Sappho's account

Pierre speaks always of meta-topics, of the true topic behind what we speak of. Grace too takes the word theme, with great emphasis. "There is a theme here. What is the theme?" So I too search for this morning's theme or meta-topic, which I am certain is the final goodbye to the leader. Absolutely, his funeral took place this morning, and life goes on for the group. The father is dead, and we are no longer children depending on him. If he comes, he comprehends or he does not; it is his problem. This account is only for the education of the group members, and of myself, of course.

Today I am more myself than before. I put my love-troubles back in Athens. My heart opens more and truly I hear more clearly what people say. I am competent again, I think. The group is warming up.

Manfred continues to be difficult. He sent a message by Birde that he was not interested in dreams, so would come to the group later. No negotiation, no direct statement. I told Birde that she was collusive to be the courier for this rude message, and that I refused to spend time as last night, worrying over his absence. It

The dream of leadership 61

is a power-play which we join in if we spend our time to make clever interpretations of why he is not here. I said also that as a systems-theorist he must know that a sub-group of one has little influence. Annie said I was beginning to do what I said we should not do. But I needed to add also that the terms of his being here are to make family therapy on us, and we do not need it. Annie's attacks on me as a younger woman need no explanation.

After a pause, Sohan told a dream which he says he has many times. It is of a tiger killing Sohan's brother, then seizing his mother. Sohan wants to save her, but his mother says he must be a good boy.

Annie had dreamt of trying to build a house of dominoes, but one was missing, so the house always fell down.

Grace and Birde also told dreams, but I have forgotten them.

Chuck told a wonderful dream of "singing up" (Chetwin 1987) his cousins on a sheep station, and hearing stories from an aboriginal worker that he could no longer remember or understand, though he wanted to. Also, Chuck dreaded his uncle, and would not sing him up, knowing he had done something very bad. This is to me a clear dream of early sexual abuse, which I have been studying on a course this Easter. Chuck eagerly assented to my offer of a full psychodrama. I walked arm in arm with him round the great library, talking quietly to help him evoke more of those early scenes of his life, and the emotionality, which is culturally a difficult area for him. I demonstrated the technique of the alter ego, by using his own words, and allowing my feelings to infuse them. The blocks in him are great. So after a time I set up a first scene with some of the group as the cousins, and Pierre as the aborigine.

The group of course needs training, and Pierre began to supply a story, rather than wait for Chuck's words, and just repeat them. But he learned fast. However, the scene was again depressed and inconclusive. So I decided on more direct catharsis, and set up all the cushions on a large sofa at one end of the room. In a very fine speech I encouraged everyone present to remember the grown-ups who had been bad to them, and evaded punishment, as had happened to Chuck. I explained how they could help Chuck by finding their own rage and expressing it. The result was a vast explosion of emotion, in shouting, beating, kicking, strangling cushions, and finally many tears from many people. Unfortunately Manfred came in at the end of this scene, and in a hostile way concerned himself with a split cushion. There was much material there for his own psychodrama, as I told him quietly.

More than two hours had passed in what I have described in such a few lines. Chuck had wept a good deal, but spoke more now of his young sister, and of locking her in a barn where she had then cut herself on a scythe. I made a summing-up story as I sat down beside Chuck, of a lost little boy sent to a strange family for the summer, of his trying to be a big man like his cousins, trying to understand strange and incomprehensible ways, like those of the old aboriginal.

"Then I guess I made a profession of it," he said at one moment, making the connection between psychiatry and that early experience. It is of course not surprising that we did not go directly to the sexual material.

I put a chair beside him and invited people, in the classic way, to sit on it in turn and tell how the experience of the morning had evoked things in their own life. Again, I had to check them from interpreting. But no one gave advice, at least. And the material evoked was enough for a productive week of psychodrama on early family themes.

My judgement was to move straight to work with Manfred, and I opened the path for that to take place. He refused. The atmosphere was electric, and I felt anger towards Annie when she said we needed a break for coffee. This is so British, to drown all feelings, to swallow them sip by sip in tea and Nescafé. But many people moved, immediately she had spoken. Grace said she would like time to ask me more about the techniques I had been using, when we returned.

During the coffee people were very quiet, wandering off alone or in pairs into the garden. I was left by myself, while Chuck went with Orminda, which troubled me. I fear a vampire in her, feasting on the dark parts of other people's lives. But I was quite exhausted, too. I have certainly not shown at all completely in this account the amount of work I put into the session. In one morning I was attempting to give a training for a whole group, and do an important psychodrama.

In the talk after the coffee I did not give so much attention all the time. Therefore I leave the tape recorder to cover what happened. We went beside the pond in the garden and lay in a circle facing inwards, all to be near the microphone.

The dream of leadership

ANNIE: In the night I woke, pregnant with such intimations of the transformations that are happening between us. Chuck's image of singing up makes me shiver. Perhaps we are just your dream too, Chuck.

ORMINDA: You're making his dream a comment about us? And I guess at Jungian images in you. You're our oceanic consciousness.

GRACE: Orminda, I wish you'd stop facilitating people. I wished you'd worked with Sappho on your own dream.

ORMINDA: I hardly had one.

GRACE: I say. Get in touch with your dream.

CHUCK: Yeah, sisters! Yeah, brothers, Ah say to you, Ah have a dream.

GRACE: Do I sound like that?

BIRDE: Yes. And I like that. It is you. You say what you want. Then I am licensed to say what I want.

SOHAN: I wish to say how much I appreciate Sappho's clear ways to explain what she does in the psychodrama. And this chance to involve many members as auxiliaries. This I should like to try with my patients. I am not assertive enough, I am very aware.

CHUCK: Not Sappho's problem. And thanks, Sapph. I got a lot out of that.

SAPPHO: And there is more to get when you are are ready. We work again.

ANNIE: Just a minute! What's going on here?

SAPPHO: You interrupt the process.

PIERRE: What process? The individualistic process of the Greek prima donna.

BIRDE: It is a Gestalt group! Speak your own response, please, not a judgement.

PIERRE: I just did, you Scandinavian—hen! I piss on you. Please. Do your thing. Do it out of my way. And I do my thing, in the immortal words of Saint Fritz of the sulphur baths. Of Saint Fritz the Promiscuous.

GRACE: I certainly see where that notion of you as a spoilt kid came from. I get dizzy when you jump from that to far-seeing interpreter, and then back.

PIERRE: Yes. I am so DESTRUCTIVE! And you all laugh.

BIRDE: I notice in my laughter, I am happy that you are big enough to be a match for Grace.

SAPPHO: I resent that I offer to do psychodrama demonstration, and you now ignore it and speak of other things.
ANNIE: I notice you are still arm in arm with Chuck, even lying here. I'm just preoccupied about therapeutic distance.
CHUCK: Am I resisting? I mean, this isn't exactly a group of patients.
GRACE: I resented your speed, Sappho, in offering to work with Chuck. I wanted some negotiation time.
SAPPHO: Thank you, Mama. I teach you now. Gestalt is the art of spontaneity.
BIRDE: I feel this attack as if on me. And with my head I can reply, spontaneity is not the same as impulse. Impulse is me-now-ignoring-much-context. Deliberation is shitting and not getting off the pot. Spontaneity is beautiful aware choice and enactment with grace. It is what Perls and Goodman call creative adjustment.
SAPPHO: Not with Grace, thank you.
SOHAN: In the night I reflect how we use the idea of the child's book, to be different animals. In the drawing exercise I think you let yourselves be art-therapy animals without reserve. But I see us resist much being Gestalt animals. Or this morning, psychodrama animals.
ORMINDA: Yes. It ain't what you do, it's the way that you do it. You are brilliant at being humble and unthreatening. So we join in. You lead by being competent too, though, I know.
SAPPHO: I too am competent.
GRACE: I think you are, very. But just so different. You lead from the front, Sappho.
PIERRE: Yes yes. Sappho is a charming dictator. Many useful therapeutic transactions may possibly happen under her dictatorship. But this is not group therapy. For group therapy, we allow. We allow the organic, irrational, inevitable but idiosyncratic processes of this particular group at this particular time to emerge. Then in these original circumstances, these novel circumstances, each member first comes to see her patterns of defence, and then perhaps experiments with new ways, finally, I must say, with new ways to live. I quote you William James (Foulkes and Anthony 1957): "*I am done with good things and big things, great institutions and big success, and I am for those tiny, invisible, molecular, moral forces that work from individual*

The dream of leadership 65

to individual, creeping through the crannies of the world like so many soft rootlets, or like capillary oozing of water, yet which, if given time, will rend the hardest monuments of man's pride."

This quotation was followed by silence.

SAPPHO: I was thinking what an intolerant group this is. So must I be humble and unthreatening, and ooze? That is not me! I feel like Manfred. That I cannot express myself here. I think I move away into the sun and get a tan.

CHUCK: You stay right here and stop being a pain in the arse. I was really getting off on that quotation, feeling real big-hearted and noble, till you started.

SAPPHO: I stay. I laugh at you and I stay.

Quiet again.

GRACE: In the silence I've kept going over the way people make a pair of me and Pierre. Gestalt and psychoanalysis. Embarrassment. The fantasy that you know a lot that I don't know gets in the way of my just insisting on Gestalt modes. That and the role confusion, with no designated leader yet.

PIERRE: It is right. Psychoanalysis knows much that is ignored or denied in these Lewinian formulations of group process. And yet, I admit, I search for new energy and ways of working, from Gestalt.

GRACE: Now I am blushing. I notice sexual images as I say, I want a fruitful marriage between us.

ANNIE: That wakens so much in me. Happy feelings that Mummy and Daddy love each other, so I need not be their little marriage counsellor. That is personal. Then behind that I suppose are all my breaking apart, fragmentation terrors, which are pregenital. Then I remember Bion's strange observations about pairing. It is a flight from the group, and the group condones it, because it also carries the Messianic promise. It symbolises the hope of continuing life (Bion 1961).

BIRDE: Now I see the so-many dimensions, the richness of each moment that you spoke of before, Annie. And for me you expressed it so clearly. And the echoes go on and outward still. With my admiration I notice competitiveness, my need to say something. And more than that. Is it all right I take a minute to say this? It pushes out of my heart and head together. I do not feel the need for victory over you, which Perls showed is finally petty, finally only self-conquest. I want to emulate, to give of my best as you seem to have done. I remember I think Alcibiades in the *Symposium* (Plato) has this idea of an army of lovers, who will each do only his best, be the best he is in the presence of the loved one. That is how I would be here.

I felt no energy in the quiet that fell again.

SOHAN: Now the building materials of Chuck's image yesterday are like inlaid marble, with precious stones carefully cut to make this shining edifice.
PIERRE: And if we look inside the shining edifice, I suppose we find the contents of Pandora's box.
ANNIE: Black and sticky. Let's stop for another coffee.
PIERRE: Black and sticky? I think you want to shit. Coffee is your British euphemism.
ANNIE: Now I see the group travelling along on all these little explosions that come from one person, then another. An internal combustion engine. Each of us has our way of galvanising the others. I suppose that is the same as leading. I feel us leading in turn in ways to do with our personalities. And those personalities have at best led us to choose our therapeutic methods. But Pierre. You seem too self-opinionated to be what I imagine as a cool analyst. God, now I'm blushing. I feel anally intruded by things you say. Prick words. And now I have that not-in-front-of-the-children-feeling, thinking of Orminda and Sohan.
SOHAN: I asssure you, I am married man with two lovely daughters already.
BIRDE: No! You're so young.
SOHAN: Excuse me. I think it easier for us to think of my youthful looks than of strange idea Annie expresses.
SAPPHO: Later. I do want a shit. And some more coffee.

Some people were away more than five minutes.

CHUCK: You did it again, Sappho. You magicked us into having coffee just now, and walked out before we'd agreed a time for coming back.

The dream of leadership

GRACE: Manfred, I'm glad you're back in the group now.
MANFRED: Such polite expressions.
SAPPHO: I have other feelings, that you walk out with no message, that you leave no possibility of communicating, of negotiating.
BIRDE: What is the English? The saucepan calls the kettle black.
GRACE: Racism!
MANFRED: In what way is this racist?
GRACE: It was a joke.
MANFRED: I think below jokes is always special meaning.
GRACE: My special meaning, the one I notice anyway, was an attempt to distract attention from you, to give you some breathing space.
MANFRED: This in Gestalt is called rescuing. It is related to mother-smothering.

Silence once more.

CHUCK: Manfred certainly reduces the score rate on Dionysiac revelry and mystic insight around here. What Birde said about emulation and stuff rather than cut-throat competition was flowing through my veins, like Pierre's quote back there, sort of buoying me up, sort of making a statement of faith, I guess, about this group.
MANFRED: This I expect. That I am made the scapegoat for the failures of the group. I retire.

Certainly thoughts of Manfred filled the silence at this point.

MANFRED: So is this a meditation group, that you have this silence? I am interested to know the advances you have made in the times I am not with you.
SAPPHO: I don't believe you are interested in the least. Look at your foot poking up, and this way you scratch the side of your nose and smile.
MANFRED: So you do not reply to my innocent question? The Palo Alto School has made interesting researches into pathogenic logic. Disqualifying and mystification. Yes.
ANNIE: I struggle between reactive feelings, and my overall response to you, Manfred, which is that I believe you have things

of value to offer to us, as we have to you. You are certainly well read.

BIRDE: Another aspect of pathogenic logic from the Palo Alto school is the double bind (Selvini-Palozzoli and others 1989). I think you attempt to put many on us now, Manfred. You dismiss us if we welcome you. And you will walk out if we are angry. That is my fantasy.

MANFRED: I observe that nobody answers my simple question of what progresses you have achieved in the several hours when I was not with you.

GRACE: I want to. It's an uncomfortably good question. I've become much more aware than before of there being two general ways in which to conduct therapy groups. The groups Pierre describes are a bit like the sort of Gestalt group I run. Leadership is to some extent a vacuum. The leader sets an ethos, and covertly trains the members to initiate for themselves.

ORMINDA: That's like Rogers' way. Then there's a whole range of therapies where the leader is more clearly the group manager from moment to moment. In management theory someone wrote about organic versus mechanistic groups (Burns and Stalker 1961). It's the same. Sappho stayed central throughout Chuck's work. The Tavistock Institute taught me so much about authority and leadership (Rice 1965).

PIERRE: I wish to ask, Sappho, did you know what you wanted Chuck to discover? You discounted his story of his sister at the end. I see not why. Foulkes teaches to value all, all that is said, every silence. You censor, I think. Now, is this the method of psychodrama, or is it your personal style?

MANFRED: You have arrived at a quite elementary contradiction, I see.

BIRDE: Manfred, you are intolerable! I have been inhibiting myself, thinking how bad for you to be allowed to act out this terrible life-script in one more episode (Pearce and Cronen 1980). But I am not here to rescue you.

GRACE: In what you call mechanistic groups, Orminda, group members know the structure ahead of time. O, so they do in the organic ones, more or less. They know the time and place, and who the designated leader is. But I see such a gulf between, say, a programme of a warm-up followed by a group exercise followed by a psychodrama followed by a sharing; at the other

The dream of leadership

end there's the Gestalt or Rogerian anarchy. But it's only just struck me. Do all the groups end up the same way, anyway? Is there equifinality, all roads leading to the same Rome?

ANNIE: Your leading is emollient, Grace. You offer an important idea, and search for commonality. The function of finding it now is I think to deflect from Manfred. I needed to comment on that process.

CHUCK: So Grace is saying that it doesn't matter if I have a kind of drill-sergeant approach to group therapy, or am laid back? The group will go where it wants to.

GRACE: Robin Skynner talks about a natural history of groups, meaning just that (Skynner 1987).

ANNIE: In Gordon Wheeler's book (1991) I found for the first time that Goodman, Perls' collaborator, was a very influential writer on social change in the sixties, and dedicated to true anarchy. It was a Gestalt view, that each person taking responsibility for themselves would lead to a responsible collective, without imposed laws and so on.

MANFRED: And so we see his handiwork in the hippie culture, and we notice how little time that persisted before becoming a drug culture, an escape culture, not of leadership, but of evasion.

ANNIE: I hadn't finished, Manfred. I wanted to say, that there is a struggle for anarchy going on here. I think we all want to recognise each other and give leadership space to each other. But we are frightened of being submerged, so we also try to make a hierarchy.

PIERRE: Perhaps there will be a real wedding between Gestalt and the psychoanalytic climate of opinion. At a primal level there is a group wish for me and Grace to be the parents of this new child. That is a safe hierarchy at one level. Yet as Annie says, with such a dream come other dreads.

BIRDE: I notice guilt. I am guilty that I do not want Jan now to walk through that door, although also I shall welcome him. But also, I betray Perls if I allow this snake of psychoanalysis back into the Gestalt garden.

GRACE: I think Perls integrated psychoanalysis, and moved on, as I think the analytic school is always moving on. Perls stopped when he died. We go on. That is a group process too. We continue the dialogue.

PIERRE: But not till later. It is lunch time.

SAPPHO: Oui, Papa.
SOHAN: I assure you it is of no importance at all to me to be the leader here. I am most happy to learn, to follow.
ORMINDA: It's a horrible idea, of Pierre and Grace as king and queen. It's atavistic. It's un-Gestalt. I just hate it.
GRACE: What's going on in you? You sound so passionate.
ORMINDA: I think ... it's to do with restoring balance.
CHUCK: If we had to have a king and queen, that pair might do pretty well. Grace'd take care of Pierre's despotic leanings. I guess you're a kind of a democratically ambitious despot, Pierre. But life sort of needs to be on your terms.
SAPPHO: Like Manfred. There is another of these caring persons who is totally autocratic. Be cared for in my way or I am hysterical, they say.
ANNIE: Is there a projective element in there, Sappho?
SOHAN: I think we go too fast.
ORMINDA: Manfred, are you going? O, he evidently was. You know, if we cannot make this place safe for him, we are leading badly.
ANNIE: That is your kind of leadership, Orminda. What Birde and Grace call holding the wide gestalt. You look at the system.
BIRDE: You are saying that Manfred is a function of the field, and we are the field. I forget this often. I think I lead like Sappho, from a great heart and some competence in the craft of one-to-one work.
CHUCK: Annie's style is to give an example of real close attention and tracking. But you're a poet, you just translate what you see into images and passion. That's more anarchic than a lot of us. I mean I guess if I was leading I'd just kind of put up a flip chart and do a brainstorm session. Late twentieth-century clever dick. OK, I observe the fidgets and I heard Annie's tummy rumble. Back here at four o'clock?
BIRDE: Our good Gestalt pupil! He speaks from observable data, even if he does not admit his own feeling and prejudice. Under the big tree at four o'clock?
SOHAN: That will be a very beautiful setting.

The dream of leadership

Jan's comment

A paradox I remembered anew as I read Sappho's report is the way power systems sometimes camouflage intimacy systems within them, and vice versa. Roger Harrison has written on the taboo subject of love in the organisation. Sonia March Nevis (with J. Zinker, 1981) is illuminating on the subject of power within the family. Therapists are right to pay attention to power games in the apparent intimacy system of individual or group therapy.

This group shifts between working as a power and an intimacy system. As an intimacy system, as when Orminda told her story, need is recognised, and the rest of you, by and large, responded as environment to that need. As a power system, different members impose themselves on the rest, dominating by affective means, as Sappho sometimes has, by taking space, as you all have at different moments, by showing sapiental authority, as many of you have from time to time, or even, like Manfred, by withdrawal.

Configuring all these episodes as political may illuminate the important power play that is around. Despotism, democracy, meritocracy and anarchy have all appeared. And the task of the group is stated as a search for what could be called a reconciliation, a melding of authorities. What is still missing in this acephalous gathering is an agreed methodology for the task.

One struggle still seems to be between therapies. This is illusory. It is between people. For example, Sappho is an, albeit benevolent, despot as a psychodramatist. This is more to do with her temperament than her discipline: Moreno was passionately interested in mobilising the initiative of group members (Greenberg 1974).

In this gathering of informed people, new ways of exercising authority are needed. The rotating leadership mooted the first evening sounded a convenient, though avoidant, structure. But so far, the group are settling for the more taxing Gestalt solution of anarchy, the authority of each one. You have not found any form or norm which will bring Manfred alongside the rest.

Finding a structure which is an adequate configuration of time, sorts of people, environment and task, needs to be an aware, even a laborious, process. In many groups it is side-stepped by the imposition of an off-the-peg, remembered structure. There are many that would no doubt be a good-enough solution here. So I admire that you expose yourselves to what may be a longwinded and emotional exercise, of enlarging your repertoire of group structures. To me it is a proper task for therapists. Politics are too crucial to be left all to the politicians. What you are doing is a contribution to achieving a responsive and responsible citizenry. It is a task seldom addressed. So this seemingly small episode of political invention is touching to me as I read about it, and imagine the skills you are giving yourself this week, even if you screw up.

If the fool persists in his folly, he will become wise (Blake).

References

Bion W. (1961) *Experiences in Groups and Other Papers*. London: Tavistock.

Burns, T. and Stalker, G. (1961) *The Management of Innovation*. London: Tavistock.

Chetwin B. (1987) *The Song-Lines*. London: Jonathan Cape.

Foulkes S. and Anthony E. (1957) *Group Psychotherapy—The Psycho-Analytic Approach*. Harmondsworth: Penguin.

Greenberg I. (1974) *Psychodrama*. New York: Behavioural Publications.

Handy C. (1991) *The Gods of Management*. London: Business Books.

Moreno J. (1946) *Psychodrama*. Beacon, NY: Beacon House.

Nevis S. and Zinker J. (1981) *The Gestalt Theory of Couple and Family Interaction*. Working paper, centre for Study of Intimate Systems, Gestalt Institute of Cleveland.

Pearce W. and Cronen V. (1980) *Communication, Action and Meaning. The Creation of Social Realities*. New York: Praeger.

Rice A.K. (1965) *Learning for Leadership. Interpersonal and Intergroup Relations*. London: Tavistock.

Selvini-Palozzoli M., Cirillo S., Selvini M. and Sorrentino A. (1989) *Family Games, General Models of Psychotic Processes in the Family*. New York: W. W. Norton.

Skynner R. (1987) In: J.R. Schlapoborsky (Ed.), *Explorations with Families, Group-analysis and Family Therapy*. London: Methuen.

Wheeler G. (1991) *Gestalt Reconsidered*. Cleveland: Gestalt Institute Press.

Chapter 6

Tuesday afternoon: Where do I belong?

Jan writes: My sense of this session is markedly different from the last. Perhaps you people have felt a gap, a missing element of scientific spirit. Now you seem to achieve between you that mix of tentativeness, intuition, excitement and scepticism which makes for the honing of data into knowledge or wisdom. It seems like you work as a team, contributive as well as idiosyncratic, self-rewarding and social, all at a time.

How well I recognise the vast difference of mood and content from one meeting of a group to another. These disjunctions are sometimes avoidant. More often they seem to take up a neglected theme, and so build towards a fuller whole life for the group. So it seems here. That obscure organising function which Goldstein described as a hierarchical tendency seems to work. What is most pressing emerges first into awareness and action. The need organises the field.

Orminda, who does the writing up, probably has something to do with this process. Like many Irish people, she speaks vividly, seeming to live into what she is saying. Much of the meeting is to do with the revealing of enthusiastically held, or generated, ideas.

In part, too, she makes the account a revealing personal essay. I speculate whether she, and others, are using the write-ups to rehearse or to avoid what they may later say in the group. She combines her own insights with a useful naivety towards some Gestalt terms. Some of what she questions has lately become a matter for debate among many Gestalt practitioners. She puts a title to her account, and it is one I can easily accept. Perhaps the "organism" that is more easily trusted now is the composite of nine groups in the nine perceptions of you people. Or eight of you, anyway: a critical mass.

Orminda's account

Trust the organism

We met as we had planned, all of us including Manfred, on time, even Sappho only five minutes late. I heard myself say that I would write up this session. It was what Gestalt calls a figure out of an empty ground, which I saw commented on in *The Gestalt Journal* (Yontef 1992). I have no idea why I said it, but I felt secure that it was right, I was right.

Then in the time before supper I sat for 38 minutes in front of an open laptop, staring at the dateline, breathing fast, thinking, imaging, furiously and incoherently, and not putting another keystroke on the screen. And me a journalist on a national newspaper for two years before I went in for teaching.

Then Grace came on me where I had hidden behind the summerhouse in the little paved garden, and she gave me the trust-the-organism line I have used as a heading. She said I organise with the whole organism, that that's what the word means. So OK, OK, as Chuck would say. And I notice how I am already taking on speech patterns from most of the group. Introjection. Swallowing whole. Grace and Birde are even having an effect on how I think.

What I have not chewed through yet is a whole uneasiness, and a good deal of excitement too, left over from yesterday afternoon and the meeting with that other group. It was too like being home again, the two opposed groups, and the Government in the form of the absent owner telling us to play nicely together. Then I see the hologram one stage down, another magnification in a Mandelbrot set (1988). Jan is the absent government of this group, and we are the citizens who so easily are at war, in spite of our grand aspirations towards harmony.

I spiral down into the atoms that make each one of us, and see that these worlds keep going, that enough good meetings are spun

Where do I belong?

out of the ephemeral matter there, to keep the show on the road. So does it matter that Manfred will spin out of our group? For that was the news he gave us. Put another way, does it matter that he ceases to exist for us, having never met us properly? Yes, it does to me.

He told us halfway through the meeting that he has to meet his wife in London on Thursday, and will then return to Germany. The feelings in me are so primitive. I want to murder him for that betrayal, and for the walking off last night with the enemy group, and spending time with them after lunch today. I see a lance sharpened brittle thin on its point and two blades, and imagine plunging it through his back. Kill him. I mutter it.

The explanations come tumbling fast from the supportive psychotherapy file. I come from a killing culture, and have suffered deaths from it without having any revenge.

If I had to choose a lover out of this lot, my neurotic choice, my unerring, rescuing, self-punishing choice would be Manfred. He combines just the arrogance and egotism and vulnerability of Michael himself. What saves me is not just that he is incapable, but that I am. I am as an individual no more than a murderous eunuch. All my love has moved out to work at a systems level, holding our group together, and seeking to get past this wall of hostility between our group and the next one.

Perhaps a group is a caricature of an individual, progressively less subtle as it gets larger. But now I want to tell some of the particular of the afternoon session.

We are acquiring a character and habits. One new acquisition was enthusiasm for the tape recorder. Instead of the wrangles at other sessions, the discussion was only about the best microphone, and our relation to it in order to be heard clearly. I have heard no worked-out discussion about this: there is just a sudden consensus. I feel it in my heart as a warm pride in the artefact of our record. It is precious, unique, a rich source or mine for all of us. And for me it already has a nostalgic quality, as, like a child, I begin to dread change, and the awful time when there is not this group. I want the bumble-bees big as grizzly bears to go on for ever bumping through the mists of blue catmint, and in and out of the climbing roses, and to hear Sappho laughing her excitement laugh on the tennis court, and see Annie through the archway, sitting on a stone seat writing her diary.

Following Pierre's talk of disclosure, we have begun too to spend time at the beginning of each session, recalling what is still figural for us from the time since we last met formally. Annie said how co-operative and quick people were at domestic chores, and that Sappho was the only person who had not helped wash up or prepare food. Sappho gave a rather muddled reply about feminist values and her individual needs. Then Grace chipped in some Marxist grit, asking what Sappho was prepared to contribute. If we were to respond to each according to their need, Grace suggested, then we needed to be clear that we were getting from each according to her ability. Sappho said she had led the whole morning and written it up. Then Annie pointed out that Birde had done the same the first night, but had also walked down to the village next morning to get the papers. Chuck rode in on a white charger at this and swept Sappho up. He does this to a lot of women. I thought he had done it to me once or twice today, in a way that meant sexual interest in me. But I think it is Sappho he fancies.

It was probably about then that Manfred said one of his disastrous backhanded remarks, something about hearing from Maurice, a member of the other group, of course, that Grace had written a history of humanistic psychology which had had very favourable reviews. He added that humanistic psychology was a very limited approach, but that it had its place. Birde shrieked at Grace,

"Say something! Do not allow him such words!" But Grace just said that what was figural for her was that Manfred was here, and contributing. We all went quiet, and I guess that others were in the same struggle as me, about whether to shout at Manfred, and in so doing, probably fall into a role he is unawarely priming us to fulfil. I began to have a different fantasy, that he lurks round therapeutic groups, secure that people will inhibit themselves in just this way. I began to warm to Sappho, who flared her nostrils and directed looks of great loathing at the problematic Berliner, while jigging her foot in a way that spoke of vicious kicks.

So many outsiders in this group. Manfred must have lived through the Berlin Airlift, when the place was an enemy-girt island kept going by that unlikely act of charity. Grace is an anomaly, black in a North European culture. I am a British outsider, a representative of an 800-hundred year old historical embarrassment. Sohan

Where do I belong?   77

is more than a third of the world away from his own language, his own culture. Annie is making herself an outsider to her training. And from this personal iconoclasm or political happening, we search to make an inside, a coherent group.

Most of us struggle to overcome our difficulties of contact within the group. We move our hostility to the boundary of the group itself, and scotomise the out-group, scotomise much of the field in which we operate. We do not look often enough for what Bateson (1979) calls *the pattern that connects*.

I tried to express some of this. It is not enough to make this group well-functioning within, between person and person. Unless we find how to Mandelbrot upwards to the next magnitude, to group with group, discipline with discipline, institution with institution, the personal turn-on is irrelevant. Pierre said that Tavistock group theory had addressed this question for many years (Miller and Rice 1967). But he did not say how, and nobody asked him.

What I had felt so urgently came out in words that sounded commonplace, and I was deflated. To defend myself, I said that Gestalt theory seemed not to cover anything about inter-group behaviour. Once more it was Grace who put me right (Merry and Brown 1987).

Sohan said that, like me, he felt great ignorance about Gestalt. He could understand what a figure meant. But he did not really understand about ground and field. Birde said that was simple, but then she got stuck in her answer and blushed. Manfred's smile tightened, as other people murmured and laughed, seeming embarrassed at their own confusion. I had not even noticed until now that I was confused too. As so often, Grace supplied:

"I guess a lot of the time, people say ground and field with much the same meaning. Some days I do. But if I think clearly, I make this distinction. The field is the whole thing, from which I am indivisible; so it is figure and ground. Lewin (1951) used the term with most authority of any writer I know, and he referred to the meaning of the word in physics. A field in physics is a bounded affair, and I think of it like an area with sheep hurdles round it, sort of movable boundaries. The oval of vision is another obvious image of a field, though it is easy to forget the organism, the subject, that is part of it. A theoretical biologist, talking about form and efficiency, shows that the structural design of living things proves to be the inverse of a physical stress diagram in terms of the anticipated load (Thompson 1952). That gives me a notion, even at a physiological level, of the indivisibility of organism and field."

"I see a contradiction," said Pierre.

"Boring, boring," said Sappho, but Grace looked straight at him in her open way, and struggled to answer. Pierre went on: "I refer to Perls' or Goodman's constant and most inelegant reference to organism and environment. Now I take it that the environment is the not-organism, the other, the outer world? In this case the field is as you describe it. But the ground of action, of what you Gestaltists call contact, is learning from personal experience. So when I take this rather pedagogic tone and demonstrate to you that I have read your texts in some detail, I am using a contact strategy, what I would call a defence against some threats you represent to me. I play the schoolmaster who was my father. That is the ground from which the present contact attempt emerges. In other words, the field is inside me."

"Now the ground has changed for me," said Grace, blushing up so she turned quite dark. "I want to know what threat I represent to you. My interest in you is the figure, against a ground of interest in our two theories."

"I think this is nonsensical," said Manfred, quite animated with bad feeling. "Please kindly to state what then is the field as you term it?"

"The field is this group," said Grace softly, looking at Pierre all the time, though he looked away now. "It is this group as it illuminates, as we illuminate, the needs and gaps and the gratifications in my whole life. It is this group as the present arena, the temporary system where I take in parts of you as Kohut (1977) describes. This is the field of which I am part, in which I am nourished and grow and which I affect and change."

"But where do you belong? Where is your reference group? The answer is most important for the psychological health," said Manfred. "It is mere romanticism to lurch from one temporary system to another, making always these dreadful contacts as you call it in Gestalt, like so many pieces of electrical wire. What is needed is the place to belong."

"And where do you belong?" asked Chuck. But Manfred did not reply. I was frightened of another men-as-intellectuals subgroup re-establishing, as Annie probably was, as she interrupted quickly. But Manfred raised his voice and talked her down: "So do you belong in your family, or your work-group, to your town or your football team or your country or university or to Europe or to a library or to what?"

"Yes," said Chuck.

"Yes to what?"

"Yes to all of them and a lot more. I'll have a badge made: I Can Tolerate Multiple Membership." Annie spoke again, and this time was listened to, or at least not interrupted. At first I imagine that several of us were preoccupied as to whether Manfred would tolerate even temporary membership of this transient system if it involved him being teased and in fact quite devalued. I really like Chuck. The tape is not clear here, but I recall more or less what Annie said:

"Last year I worked on an Open University Summer School for two weeks. It was very exhilarating, and very new, all those people eagerly thinking and questioning. I hardly slept, for nights and nights. Then just near the end of the time, I woke in the early hours one morning, and had a most strange experience. It was not a vision, because there was nothing visual about it at all. It was tactile, if anything, though that is not a good description either. In retrospect, it seemed a sort of pre-verbal glimpse. I don't suppose it lasted more than about four seconds. But it just stays with me, informs me. The only bad thing about it is that every time I have tried to tell people about it, they have ignored me or changed the subject or just misunderstood. I want to tell it now. May I?"

"It is you who will give the permission," said Birde, being her usual dependable Perlsian Gestalt stereotype. Annie continued:

"I had the sense of waking into slowed time. I'm reducing what happened by translating it into words. But that is the only language between us now. It was as if everything was moving, like a dark kind of dough kneading itself. In that inexorable movement was everything that has ever happened to me, and to all that went before me, right back to the unwelded atoms and bits of stars from which we are made. The dough was all that, and the learning I had made out of each experience. And out of all that, inevitably, the next I Need or I Want, the next impulse to my next action in the world was coming to the surface of awareness, if I bothered to notice. That's all it was. It's probably the most important experience I have ever had. And then about a month later someone explained Gestalt therapy to me, and it seemed very near what I had felt through my whole body or self or whatever the word is."

"Like a blinding light on the road to Damascus, except that it was an enlightening dark," said Grace. I could see that she had said the right thing for Annie. Even Sappho co-operated with her: "By this you construct your meaning, you see that the field is a combination of what is already within the self, and what can be internalised in the moment of the outer world?"

"It made me see the extraordinary importance of every single moment and, in the ordinary phrase, what I make of it. I am always always always shaping my capacity to handle the world, or, put another way, my life," said Annie.

Grace added quietly, "In Gestalt words, you are always affecting your response-ability, your ability to respond. I think that is what Perls meant when he talked about the self as the contacting."

Pierre fidgeted and cut across what she was saying. "You do not understand all you are saying, neither you nor Annie. This is a definition of the self as the sum, or the whole as more than the sum of the part" ... here he saluted as if to some God of Gestalt... "of the totality of this organism of which you Gestaltists speak. In this definition the now is clearly the product of all that has gone before. It incorporates the totality of the past, and even as much of the future as can be postulated by this organism in this state of learning."

"You are going too quickly," said Birde. Pierre turned to her and continued:

"It is very clear, and very profound. If self is to be a function rather than an image, as Perls recommends, then it will be a function—or no, rather it will be *the* function—of an integrated whole, not of some small department of the organism called a contact boundary or some other term quite devoid of humanity or grace."

"Me again," said Grace, grinning at him, "You keep bringing me into the conversation."

"This you say from your now, from your self, in this vocabulary. The coincidence with my now has to be explored," said Pierre. Grace changed tack:

"As I said, Lewin spoke of the oval of vision sighted people have. He used it as an illustration of the limitation of field we impose on the world, without noticing. But it is a simplistic idea,

Where do I belong? 81

compared with this rich idea or experience that Annie offers us. From what she says I think we can construct a unified theory." Annie was not listening.

"To go on with that oval of vision image: it is not just what my eye lights on," said Annie, "it is the capacity I have achieved to make whatever sense I do of what I see or hear or experience in any way, that is the key to who I am, and therefore to what I am likely to do to you. I am always your environment, affecting you."

"Psychodrama is very clear in this," said Sappho. "The protagonist is the figure, and the auxiliaries are the ground. But always in flux. All are in turn protagonists. And so the field enlarges while we witness, to allow into the experience of all, the deep life experiences and struggles and changes in each."

"That helps me a lot," said Chuck. "So I could say, the field in a psychodrama group at one moment would include the problem just recounted, say, by one group member, plus the selves, the life-experience, of everyone present, and the amount of attention and insight available in their 'now', and then the ordinary constraints of the size of the room and what time the group has to break, and stuff like that. The protagonist is the figure in the ground of the surrounding auxiliaries and the director."

"The figure shifts in gestalt formation, through fore-contact, contact, final contact. There's always the Heraclitan flux, not a fixed figure," said Grace.

"O my God," said Sohan, "Never have I been buffeted by so many large ideas in so little time. My heart beats and I am all questions. But also I am aware that we do not yet decide our arrangements for the evening session."

"I feel full. Can I tolerate another session?" said Annie, doubtfully.

"Yes yes," said Birde, "there is so little time. Already we approach the halfway of the group."

"If I don't dance I die," said Sappho. I found that I agreed with each of them as they spoke. At the same time I was exhausted, over-stimulated and needing thinking time, and frightened of being alone, or perhaps being cornered by Birde and stuck in a desultory conversation about drunkenness in Sweden, as happened at lunch. Chuck looked at the floor and did not speak. I realised that I wanted to do what he would do; but I too kept quiet. Pierre said that if we met it should be to continue this most interesting seminar, but explicitly to avoid emotional material. Grace asked Manfred his opinion. He said the sun was in his eyes. She said we could move. He said the sun would move again. She said that it seemed as if we were ending the group anyway, and that she had asked about his evening preference.

"I have decided," he said grandly, "I spend time with some most cultivated persons from the barn group." Poor Manfred. He seems to have learned only how to behave as a human hedgehog. And we have not found a way to let him uncurl.

Sappho and Birde certainly administered a few verbal kicks to him at this point, and Chuck stared through him.

"But you're leaving on Thursday, Manfred," said Grace. "And I don't feel we've got through to you yet."

"Perhaps I do not wish to be got through to," said Manfred coldly.

"You said it, brother," said Chuck. Grace changed the subject, saying, "I'm not clear about having a group or not having a group tonight. Let's meet in the library at half past eight to decide."

Jan's comment

Earlier, you seemed at moments to be a collision of nine worlds. Now, as I said, there is far less scrapping and scrambling for position. Sohan's difficulty with some Gestalt terms is made into an opportunity for everyone to try and hone their sense of what certain words mean. Staying with the thoughts of Daniel Stern (1985) that I have often had as I read, it looks like you are as a group beginning to use the verbal self as a tool to enlightenment, rather than a neurosis-maker. And the limitations of words are acknowledged by Annie when she recounts her vision or mystic experience. In Buber's (1958) term, many other group members *include* her: they see the world from her point of view, rather than contesting it from theirs. In terms of contact boundaries, they let in what she is saying, to illuminate their own experience and thoughts. Then they communicate again, so the illumination grows as a co-creation. Parts of the session are an exemplum of this desirable and seldom-sustained way of conversing. Within it, Annie dares to tell what seems an aware glimpse of a massively important evolutionary process.

Annie's description is to me a wonderful illumination of Gestalt *responsibility*. I am responsible for what I do with every interaction with you, as for everything I do in the world. My actions will seep or ricochet out through the present, into the physical world, and down through the generations. Detectives say contact leaves trace. Always. Boy, that's immortality. That's more power than it's comfortable to contemplate.

And the beautiful thing that happens here is that for the first time Annie feels heard when she tells her vision. Other people in the group take in what she says, and expand or reinforce her meaning for her. Carrying a belief all alone is lonely, unnatural and can get a little mad. Even the story of the life of the Buddha is a story of a co-operation towards enlightenment by many spirits and people. In our group, openness breeds openness. Orminda even tells secrets about herself in the writing up.

She also reveals an anxiety that things should go well, and a fear of dissension. Maybe that is what leads to the strange non-responsiveness of Manfred after a time. I began to guess that the group kind of paints him out for much of this meeting. Maybe the way you do acknowledge him is by showing how collaborative you can be—not with him, but with each other. Whether this is meant to reassure him, or is a more hostile display, I can only guess. Every tool can be a weapon; this would not be the first time I have suspected that even harmony can in part be used as an offensive weapon. Manfred's insistence on the importance of the reference group gets the scant attention that often follows his interventions. There is a considerable possibility that many of you lack secure reference groups, and do rely on transient work groups of students and patients, for some of your sense of belonging. It seems it is hard for the rest of you to hear someone who so often sounds attacking.

For most of you, it seems like you have relaxed into trust, and really gotten to listening. Even reading this, I noticed my neck and shoulders loosen, and my mind went wider. No way does it surprise me that multi-membership is being acknowledged now. Exploring Gestalt terms seems a tacit recognition that people can belong here, as well as hold membership of the psychoanalytic or family therapy or psychodrama school. The confidences I mentioned earlier are another product of and process towards a sense of belonging here.

What are the forces that have brought about this beginning of a shift? Manfred has probably influenced a closing of ranks, as has the meeting with the counselling group. You now have some shared history, both in the sense of things you have done together, and in the sense of self-revelation by words. Fibre by fibre, glance by glance, response by response, you have provided enough of you with enough data, it seems, to decide that you can let go more, and move towards excitement and growth, rather than defensiveness and conservatism. Everything counts. Make no mistake, you have counted everything. In Stern's words, you have made from them RIG's, Representations of Interactions you have Generalized (Stern 1985, p. 97). And there is part, I guess, of the bad feeling around Manfred. Is it that he is incapable of reading you all? Or are you really not worth the time of this gifted and tetchy fellow?

Orminda's own ideas about gaining skills at meetings between groups and in large groups becomes open. This group is perhaps dependable enough for enough of you to let you look beyond its boundaries.

Awareness and tolerance of belonging to many groups is a recognition of reality. It is also a powerful force towards social harmony. I think of recent history: while Europe struggled to hold its EC member states together, countries such as Iraq and the former Yugoslavia have shown murderous intolerance of the idea of belonging to a nation as well as an ethnic group. Denying connectedness can be a sure path to hostility.

The paternoster lift continues, dredging from below awareness up into awareness, and returning new material to shape what in Perls' terms perhaps becomes physiological (Perls, Hefferline and Goodman 1951).

You are opening boundaries to what is inside as well as outside, to the apparent polarities of going deeper into the intrapersonal and more enlightenedly into considerations of larger systems, almost at the same time. It is as if the contact-boundaries between people have become osmotic for more or even most of the time. Now, the whole is not so often being preserved for each member by excluding what is perceived as alien or invasive. Growth is happening, as you work to let in, rather than keep out. As you may have guessed, I am back with my political analogies. You, or we, have a lot to teach politicians. And I think we have things to learn from them too.

Where do I belong?

How angry I am that I can only read about what I would so dearly have loved to be part of! A major theme started here, and continued from now, is the notion of aware heterogeneity. The illusion of singleton status (Turquet 1975) has yielded to a sense of many memberships, all of which form the member in some way. The way these memberships are tuned in and out of awareness has profound consequences in behaviour, as the next session begins to show.

Do you remember the Law of Praegnanz? Kohler (1927) states in essence that there is a psychological organisation of data, related to proximity, simplicity, stability and closure, and to a kind of simplifying out to as good, as clear a gestalt as conditions allow. From the mass of material generated in this group, there seems in this session to be a synchronistic decision that people have value for each other, and the Gestalt mode has value too.

With only slightly different strength of field forces, the simplification might have been that the leaderless group was not working and should disband. So each and every intervention has had its importance in creating the climate in which this organisation of data, this present gestalt, is emerging.

It is as if the music has gone slower and quieter, after much trumpeting and tympany in earlier sessions. There is much more acceptance of each other among members. We shall never know whether, say, accepting Gestalt ideas is merely an available symbol of expressing a move towards harmony, or whether the intrinsic worth of the ideas, like the intrinsic worth of Annie's vision, brings the harmony into being. When I let myself belong to a group and its ideas and values, I like to think that the latter explanation is right. I need to remind myself that I may sometimes or always be merely rationalising a pre-verbal, a non-verbal impulse to approach and ally. Manfred reminds me of the exile in the Anglo-Saxon poem, *The Wanderer* (Sweet 1876). The sense of belonging has seemed too much of a threat for him to tolerate. To the rest of you, it seems to be glowing up like a summer sunrise, with all the promise of warmth to come.

References

Bateson G. (1979) *Mind and Nature: a Necessary Unity*. New York: Dutton.

Buber M. (1958) *I and Thou*. New York: Scribners.
Kohler W. (1927) *The Mentality of Apes*. New York: Harcourt, Brace.
Kohut H. (1977) *The Restoration of Self*. New York: International Universities Press.
Lewin K. (1951) *Field Theory in Social Science*. New York: Harper Brothers.
Mandelbrot. In: Gleick J. (1988) *Chaos—Making a New Science*. London: Heinemann.
Merry U. and Brown G. (1987) The Neurotic Behaviour of Organisations. New York. Gardner Press.
Miller E. and Rice A. (1967) *Systems of Organization*. London: Tavistock.
Nevis E.C. (1987) *Organisational Consulting: A Gestalt Approach*. New York: Gardner Press.
Perls F., Hefferline R. and Goodman P. (1951) *Gestalt Therapy. Excitement and Growth in the Human Personality*. New York: Julian Press.
Stern D. (1985) *The Interpersonal World of the Infant*. New York: Basic Books.
Sweet (1876) *Anglo-Saxon Reader*. Oxford University Press.
Thompson D'A. (1952) *On Growth and Form*. New York: Cambridge University Press.
Turquet P. (1975) Threats to identity in the large group. In: L. Kreeger (Ed.), *The Large Group: Dynamics and Therapy*. London: Maresfield Reprints.
Wheeler G. (1991) Gestalt Reconsidered. New York: Gardner Press Inc.
Yontef G. (1992) Considering *Gestalt Reconsidered*. In: *The Gestalt Journal* **15**: 105.

Chapter 7

Tuesday evening: The group beast

Jan writes: If I had been there.... But I was not. And I am more bothered than I want to be, by the role some of you give me in that strange story-telling episode at the start of your evening.

The shift to the middle phase of violent happenings is startling. I put the words Group Beast in the heading. The verbal goes to the wall, and the bodies take over. Less pretty. More informative. So the ending of the evening seems the rounding of an important gestalt which has been elbowing its way into awareness over days. The path of excess has finally led to the palace of wisdom, like I said (Blake 1794). The group moves from lowly worm, via cock of the walk, to something nearer human.

And I notice that I talk of the group now as if it is an entity, rather than a composite. That is the theme I would like to take up in my final comments on the evening. It looks to me as the sessions move on, as if in most respects you make enough commentary on yourselves as you go along.

Annie's account

I have noticed that someone who is very active or influential in a session takes responsibility for writing it up. Or perhaps it is that anyone who undertakes to write up a session, then becomes something of a star, or at least a very active participant.

The thought comes to me, that my writing up the session now

is a kind of thanks to people for listening so enlightenedly to my old vision this afternoon.

I will stop asking questions, and tell what I remember of the evening.

Over supper there was a lot of discussion of Gestalt theory. If only my students would put themselves as hard at whatever they are supposed to study, how short we could make training courses!

Manfred said that Gestalt has no developmental theory, I remember (Tobin 1990). It was a relief for me that he said it, as I have thought the same. Birde said that Perls' oral aetiology of the neuroses amounted to a developmental theory. Then she herself gave a heretical admission, saying that Gestalt for her lacked a spiritual dimension. Grace then came down on her, pointing out, as far as I remember, that by splitting off spirituality as a separate entity, Birde was being un-Gestalt. If mind and body are indivisible, then so is spirituality implicit in them. Again, I was reassured. Jungian analysis has been so freeing for me, allowing as it does the sense of the cosmic, the archetypal, the spiritual.

I do not want to devalue that, if I begin to work in a more Gestalt way. People spoke too of my mystic experience or whatever it should be called. I think that may have given me the confidence, once we had all settled in the library, and pulled the sofas and armchairs into some kind of circle, to tell the story which seemed to be waiting in me to be uttered. A chilly wind and a rainstorm had come up just before supper. That made more of a story-telling atmosphere.

ANNIE: Once upon a time there was a band of pilgrims. No. It was a band of philosophers. They came over land and sea to find other philosophers who would understand the complexity of their thoughts, and the simplicity and goodness of their beliefs. In their own lands in their own ways they had helped many people to find their own wisdom and use it in their lives. But when the philosophers met, they encountered a strange magic. He who for that time was to be their leader was missing. In a silent ritual, without noticing what they were doing, the philosophers immediately knelt down and made to him a propitiary sacrifice of their own great powers. In this way they put on themselves the curse of fear; they knew that whoever among them held sway over the rest might be torn to pieces and made

The group beast

as nothing. They were aghast to find that such fears and such envy could come upon them in the place of pilgrimage.

BIRDE: One of them turned on herself and resolved to tear herself into pieces before the others could reach her. She told herself that she was unskilled, and felt shame. She told herself that she was despicable to feel envy towards the others, and felt guilt. She told herself her own simple beliefs were naive compared with those of some of the other better-informed philosophers, and in this way she destroyed her own history, so the blood ran cold in her veins and she felt of less worth than the mud which is carried into the house on a boot.

SOHAN: O, not only one was acting in this way, I think. But this other one was trying also to make a harmony at some moments, until he was very frightened that this was a bad behaviour to be doing.

ORMINDA: And another tried also to bind the group of philosophers together, with a desperate magic, by coming naked before them. Then she saw them at times tongue-tied by pity and dread, so her nakedness made them wrap their robes tighter round themselves.

SAPPHO: One of the philosophers quickly took a robe of defiance, and another of sexuality, to make her identity. The English is difficult. Yes, also a veil of pride that she was secretly the best leader with the best training and the quickest insight and the most creative interventions. Contempt. Yes, this was also another of her seven veils to cover the nakedness which another philosopher had so simply and so overpoweringly revealed.

CHUCK: The dumbest of the philosophers had travelled the longest way to be there. That's me, folks. Half the time he didn't even notice the magic going on round him. So he did his little numbers. He's all over the bloody place still.

PIERRE: And this philosopher was a great expert in feelings of superiority. Inside his robes he at first held conversations with himself. He despised that the other people with him seemed not well to make the translation from one scene to another. And his superiority was an illusion, a great illusion, as the story shows. Because he had given in to this enchantment of concealing his knowledge.

CHUCK: I can't say I was too aware of that happening.

SAPPHO: Sh. Let him go on.

PIERRE: So as always in good fairy stories, it was the pure voice of the child asking simple questions which broke the spells invented by the pride of the clever ones. I thank you, Sohan. It is less than nothing to know something. What I do with this knowledge, how I affect the world with it, is the only measure of what I am. Yes. I learn that again here. And I speak of another philosopher, I think much like me, although he is German. But I think he has been less loved. He has less ego-strength. So all he has known how to do is punch the noses of other philosophers, and then feel self-contempt, and then to walk away, as I notice he has now. And I acknowledge again that I have not worked as I could to open a door for him to enter here.

SOHAN: Manfred told, I forgot to say, he sees again his friend now.

There was noticeable silence before Orminda spoke.

ORMINDA: Annie, thank you. That was extraordinary. You just came in and started that story, and without any scene-setting or discussion we all tuned in as if we'd learned the music in our cradles.

BIRDE: I think we had. I feel excited to be in so wonderful a group of people. Yes. I know all people are wonderful if we make the conditions for them to be so. But that does not stop these people being wonderful. There! I have unspelled—what do you say?

GRACE: Exorcised?

BIRDE: Yes, I have exorcised the Pierre-in-me.

There is an irony, that I came to this group in part to try to exorcise my tendency to be heavy and meaningful, what my ex-husband calls Ingmar Bergmanish. Have I instead just pushed everyone else into being like me?

Chuck, who was very sweet to me at supper, interrupted at this point to say he had had enough meaning for one day. Sappho was on her feet at once, brandishing a tape and saying she needed loud music. Most of the rest of us howled her down, literally, and she sat again, looking sulky. Birde fetched a tape of a circle dance, which I am afraid was a little meaningful too. We held hands in a circle and stumbled about. Birde wanted us to look into each

The group beast

other's eyes when we danced. I notice that I avoided Pierre's, but sought Chuck's. He is the only truly manly man here. As so often in such groups, there are more interesting women than interesting men.

By interesting, in this group, I realise that I mean sexually vibrant. And now all this Gestalt indoctrination makes me re-phrase that, to acknowledge that it is I who am sexually vibrant with certain people. In my new boldness of blurting, I told this, though omitting my reaction to Chuck.

I could actually experience as a body sensation the suppression of this central material, the attraction to Chuck. Mostly it was a stiffening at either side of my neck just at the base of my skull. That made a deadness down my spine, and then a familiar kind of sad lurch through my heart and down into my viscera. But the thought of telling that I was taking a sexual interest in Chuck was worse to contemplate than bearing this hidden depression.

Excitement and growth in the human personality is the sub-title of Perls' great book. I had made the opposite choice.

The recording tape had been turned off when the dance started, and was not put back on, so from here I must rely on my memory.

Birde and Chuck left the room together after the circle dance, she smiling very widely. There was a faltering in the conversation, and I was not the only woman to look across at the door rather often. Pierre, evidently noticing what was going on, began one of his angry-sounding passionate speeches about the sexualisation of affect. He was like a thin dog barking cacaphonously and ineffectively.

Chuck and Birde came back quite soon, with a tray of glasses and three big bottles of wine, which we had only this evening noticed was there in the kitchen cupboard for us to buy.

Sohan of course does not drink, but all the rest except me filled glasses, and emptied and re-filled them more quickly than I liked to see. Perhaps it was my heaviness that was being counter-balanced.

Sappho's unspeakable blaring tape was soon on, and the windows and french windows had to be stood wide as people danced and sweated and the room became stuffy. Even Sohan was dancing wildly. There was a continual shifting of pairs, and I found myself joining in competitively, to attract one of the men, even if Chuck seemed more attentive now to Orminda than to me.

Suddenly I thought, perhaps the dancing was an inter-group event. It seemed so antithetical to the bland goodwill of the counselling group in the barn, and to their several members from closed religious orders. The profane was being displayed to the sacred, whose evening lamps could be seen at the barn windows across the yard. An angry glee came up in me, and I joined in with the yells and squeals that made our dancing, except for the tunes and rhythms, reminiscent of a Scottish New Year party.

Now I see images of the Year-King and the Bacchantes tearing him to pieces after making him drunk and, so improbably, forcing him into orgiastic performances with them all. I see them in my mind as I remember Manfred walking by with a small group of the counsellors. Chuck and Sappho were in the van of our group as we rushed out of the french windows, yelling to them to join us. We linked hands and pranced round them, and there was nothing invitational in the menace of what we were doing.

And I could not even pretend that I was drunk, like several of the rest of us.

Manfred said something in a low voice to his friend Maurice the Rabbi, and they broke the circle between me and Sohan, and the counselling group ran off towards sanctuary in their own building, with us streaming after them through the dusk. The next thing I knew, Manfred was on the ground with Chuck on top of him, clutching round him with both arms, while Manfred wriggled and shouted. I heard myself scream:

"Get off, you bugger!" Even in the horror of the moment, I could see that the scene did look like buggery, and that that was probably what had made me react so violently. Chuck stood up, and Manfred scrambled out of the mud and dashed into the barn, the other group's place. We stood there quite crestfallen among the puddles, with the tape pounding away in the background.

"We must go and say sorry," said someone, I think Grace.

"We didn't mean anything," said Sappho.

"Yes," said Pierre, "we meant all of this. It is the acting out. It is unprincipled and dangerous and I wash my hands of it."

"OK, Pontius," said Chuck, "That leaves you with the moral high ground. But we've got one of our group members in trouble in there." He made it sound as if Manfred was a virgin who had been ravished by the barn tribe.

"Then someone must go inside," said Pierre. There was a

moment of quiet. The whole of this conversation was more muddled, and took longer to happen than it does to tell. We were slow and shocked. Birde said, "But who will bell the cat?"

"I will be happy to go and apologise," said Sohan. Of course. Grace pointed out the fixed-gestalt nature of this offer. There was quiet again, as we waited for Chuck to offer. When at last he did, Birde and Orminda and Sappho almost simultaneously offered to go in with him. Then one of them suggested that we all go, and for a moment this seemed the answer. But Grace again intervened, suggesting that we would look like an invading force if we all went. Pierre said that she should go with Chuck, and the two of them approached the closed door, while the rest of us waited a short way off.

Chuck put his hand on the door handle, and I could just discern Grace pull him back, and then use the door-knocker, making a suitably doleful single knock. When no-one came, I felt wrath and contempt. How dare these people spurn our overtures? Then Manfred looked out of a window and asked what we wanted.

"To apologise," said Grace.

"Yeah," said Chuck, less eloquent. Manfred did not expostulate; but he was not very willing to return with us, as Grace urged him.

"Why should he come to purge us of our guilt?" asked Pierre in a whisper to the voyeur party. We went back without him to the untidy library, where the tape had at last stopped its frenetic blare.

It was chilly, for the first time since our arrival, as we waited for Manfred to come back. This pause was at first somehow messy, with people shuffling off to fetch coffees or on unstated missions.

We were all in the room eventually, and Orminda suddenly said, "Mother of God, did you see those nuns run for their lives when Chuck came at them?" There was a huge laugh, and Birde kept giggling.

Chuck changed the mood for the rest of us, saying he did not know what had hit him. I wanted to say that it was Manfred who was in that state, but I contained the thought. Chuck went on:

"I just went at him. I didn't even know I was going to bring him down. It was sort of horsing around." Then I revealed the sense that had gathered in me, that we were forming up for such a moment, all through the dance.

"Please," said Sohan, "I do not understand. You say we had feelings against the other group. But it was one of our group who was, who was horseplayed." I am sure he checked himself from saying the word attacked.

Grace said, "Retroflection. There's a lot of it here. Birde, Annie, Orminda, Sohan. Me too. I see most of us doing for ourselves often what would probably be better as a two-party interaction. And now this episode is a really bizarre retroflection. It looks like a parable of self-conquest (Perls, Hefferline and Goodman 1951). The other group is the defined enemy. But the brunt of this group's attack was on one of our own members."

"Who had, however, for the moment defined himself as one of them," said Pierre. "It is this that is the significant."

"Aw, come on," said Chuck, "I'm not buying that, if you're meaning it was kind of a chance that I went for poor old Manfred rather than, say, the mustachioed Maurice."

"Manfred was the over-determined object," said Pierre.

"And in Gestalt, I would translate that into the simple statement that he was carrying a lot of projections," said Grace, "Jan is another defecting male in this group that we maybe need to horseplay, as Chuck calls it. And I guess Manfred is all the part of *me* that has wondered earlier on whether to quit the group, wondered whether you were all interesting enough for me; so long as I project those ideas on to him, and wonder whether he is weighing me up and finding me wanting, I'm going to feel pretty vengeful at him."

"It is fascinating," said Pierre, "that now we define what you call the organism as the group itself. For long, it was a question of me against the rest of you. I had to maintain my defences against this group. But now we strive to maintain this group against Them, the others. We are now in misery that Manfred comes not back. We do not like him. He is insufferable. But we must have him." There was a little protest at Pierre's including us all in his pronouncements on Manfred. But everyone looked thoughtful.

Birde had stopped giggling, and said sadly, "Does there always have to be an enemy? Surely not."

"The actualities on the television will tell you the answer," said Pierre.

"It's about picking the right fights," said Grace. "It looks as if we're all agreed that this Chuck and Manfred thing was the wrong fight. I think the right one is between us and our fear. There was the fear I've talked about, that Manfred held some of the secret judgements I'd had of him, about me. And then there's the even less rational fear that the counselling group will, or could, destroy us. Steal a member. Laugh at us, as they did. Do something undefined against us. That is what I need to face: not just the actual people."

Grace is still our authority, our Jan-substitute. Orminda is the princess, the promise and glowing beauty of the group, though in fact she is not specially pretty or handsome. But her gestures have taken on more poise, hour by hour, since the racked time of her telling her story. She seems silently to have taken in and made into her own the tenderness that is the general group feeling towards her.

Here I violate Gestalt, knowingly. There is a group agreement, a turning all at one time towards a new attitude, silver-swift as a school of fish turning as one. I write it here, and will argue it aloud later. But back to the one-by-one.

Maybe Pierre's eclipse in the first part of the evening was because of the shadow of Chuck, who has been dominant male today, as I have made clear. Only now he has disgraced himself, almost as an act of self-punishment. Birde is another who is a little overshadowed, but by Grace. Grace's Gestalt seems to be more in favour than what we are learning to call Perls' Esalen Gestalt, which is what Birde knows best. She looked greyer than this morning.

Manfred at last came in through the french windows. The rest of us, after the first person had made several muddy footsteps on the carpet, had left our shoes at the door. We all watched him carry mud across the room and, as he sat, unknowingly wipe all that had been on his heels on to the frill round the bottom of his armchair. But no one told him.

Chuck, pale and tired—and drunk, I suppose—said again that he apologised. Birde repeated the word apologise, and said how remote it sounded, how unconnected with sorrow, which is what she felt. She said that when we were dancing before the incident with Manfred, we had felt to her like a carnival group, magicked into mindlessness, and being creative in new ways. Then we had turned into, she searched for a word, and Grace supplied lynch-mob, which she said was exact.

"Alone I could never intercept and taunt and tease in this way," she added. "Now I understand how crowds will kick someone to death, even. I was all elation, with no judgement."

"But I had a part in this," said Manfred, true to his systems theory. "I had gone to East Berlin and had to be punished for my inexplicable defection." Grace cradled this metaphor in her hand and offered it back to him. It was touching to see the response in him. He seemed like a hit dog who has come to heel, and is terribly eager to please and be accepted.

He told us that his grandmother and all the relations he loved best were in East Berlin through his childhood. When the wall was built, he was on the other side of it with his parents, whose bad marriage had been rendered harmless for him in early childhood by the strong extended family.

"Such a clear transference," said Pierre. "And these older kindly women in the other group..."

"And Maurice, he was as my brother who lived always with my aunts while I alone was in this torture house of my parents," Manfred interrupted. His trousers were filthy on the knees from where he had been thrown down, and I thought how we had been either the torture family, or the torture playground at school he was no doubt adept at evoking.

We spent a long and healthy time, letting him tell more of his story and feelings, and adding our honesty to them. Grace helped him to remember his successes, like his marriage, which he prizes in a way that makes me uneasy.

"I get the feeling," said Birde, "that you are letting yourself be different here at this moment, from how you might be in many situations." Manfred agreed obediently, all his grandiosity gone now. He seemed to recognise for the first time that he repeatedly sets up tests for other people, to see if they care for him.

"And the tests are all to destruction point?" said Grace. He agreed, and she went on: "And now the scene is different. You are not destroyed, and we are not destroyed."

Manfred turned suddenly towards Chuck and said, "Tell you are sorry, tell you are sorry." His voice was a high childish whine.

"I am very sorry," said Chuck gravely. I admired that he did not point out that he had already apologised twice. Birde came into her own now, and had a gentle conversation with Manfred about the origins of that demand of his. He connected it to his father's telling the family that Manfred was a coward, when he was on a picnic at a swimming pool. In reply, the four-year-old had walked out on the low diving board. His father had then pushed him in and he had nearly drowned. Most of the group joined in vicarious indignation, which he seemed to need, and then the reparative translations to the present, that Grace had begun.

Pierre put his arm round Manfred as we began at last to disperse. To my surprise, I did the same to Birde, whose one-to-one work is admirable. Till now I have felt some antagonism to her quality of, ageing sprite is the phrase that comes, and which I am tempted to censor. Then I came up to write this before falling asleep.

I have tired thoughts about our need for someone—perhaps we should call her or him a duty officer—to put in the disciplines on us that were missing in that id-level dance scene, and the hunting of the other group and Manfred. Anarchy is too taxing for me.

Jan's comment

Gestalt and group forces

In Annie's musings over group or group-mind as an entity more powerful than one individual, she is making implicit comment on an exciting and generally ignored central tension of Gestalt. Foulkes, not a Gestaltist, speaks helpfully in this area:

> It is possible to lay emphasis on the working of the group-as-a-whole (of the group as an instrument of therapy) without committing oneself to the more metaphysical view of group-as-an-organism, boasting a "group mind", a "group temperament" and, under conditions of stress, developing "group symptoms". (Foulkes and Anthony 1957, pp. 21–22)

You could argue that I-am-responsible-for-myself is a slogan at variance with ideas of, say, a collective unconscious. But Gestalt also argues the indivisibility of organism and environment. The field is unified. These notions nudge me to a suspicion that, not only do we have such overlapping evolutionary experience that we are likely to be roughly the same in many ways; too, I can believe in systems of communication between us that we use without knowing we use them. I will stick my neck out here and tell you that I have come to suppose that the same processes that result at intrapsychic level in dreams, may be responsible at group level for some of the group manifestations that surprise the people who bring them about. We signal to each other mighty fast and effectively without words, I guess. Then we are in a muddle about where the resulting actions originated.

There is a good deal of analytic theory, and rather less Gestalt, to describe many of the events of this evening. Perls was impatient with Freud's emphasis on unconscious mind, and had almost nothing to say about unconscious group dynamics. In terms of these, Chuck may have been used by the group, been the person-most-open-to-being the group's crossness with Manfred. But Annie was suspicious that the dancing earlier was an inter-group event; the group subliminally suggested and enabled the behaviour they then found Chuck somewhat unacceptable for continuing.

There must be philosophical contradictions here. But I can maintain a belief in what could be called free will, alongside recognition of the total enmeshment of every organism in its ecological field. *Everything possible to be believed is an image of truth* (Blake 1794).

What is incontrovertible is that some communication takes place, out of awareness, to license or suggest behaviours in a group that might be unacceptable to any member if alone. Thus Chuck comments his assault on Manfred. Thus riots, lynchings, witch-hunts. Thus the urgency of the Gestalt therapeutic task of raising awareness, at the level of systems much larger than the individual, or the small group *in vacuo*.

Let me deal here with the voice in me, that I project on to Manfred, I think, or even Orminda. It says that I use findings from one kind of task or group, the therapeutic, to theorise about quite other kinds. Like Bion (1961) I have a strong sense of the affective life that is inevitably there in any group. Like Bud Feder, like Zinker, like the Polsters and many other Gestalt thinkers, I believe the search for safety and trust in the group to be a sign of health. Those words, safety and trust, are ciphers to describe both the healing and the creative potential which has to be there in any group, any system, if the people who form it are to be the best of themselves within the limitations of the environment.

Therapy in its roots means service. That servicing, maintenance, affective welfare function is what entrances Annie here in much of this account, and mainly I suppose because it is so little attended to elsewhere. That is specially obvious in the case of Manfred. I can imagine a healthier society, when what we call therapy is subsumed into the work of other groups. And too, or before that, when what we call politics are addressed in therapy groups. Wow, now I feel better.

Gestalt theorists have perhaps not interested themselves overmuch in these questions since Goodman's passionate example of social vision. But the theory accounts convincingly for the change of behaviour as the environment changes. In Lewin's formulation, $B = fPE$, where B equals behaviour, P stands for person, and E for environment. He postulated the group as a dynamic whole, more easily described in terms of present vectors than in historic libidinal forces (Lewin 1936). What I need to notice is that when group membership of a present or other group is a strong influence in gestalt formation, people do things that are sublimely social or catastrophically anti-social.

Bringing to awareness the dynamics of such an incident as the rowdyism of this evening's session, could be one step towards a political survival strategy.

> Moving into the realm of healing through meeting, we must face the radical question of whether true healing, in the first instance, is not only psychotherapy, but also family, social, economic and political therapy. The readjustment of the intrapsychic sphere is a byproduct. (Friedman 1985, p. 97)

Part of that larger therapy is to get more understanding of whether a group is a mere structure, like a train you enter in order to go a journey, or whether it is a psychic entity of which you and I are no more than the expressive elements, however cunningly we bluster and rationalise to preserve our self-respect, our *amour propre*.

References

Bion W. (1961) *Experiences in Groups*. London: Tavistock.
Blake W. (1794) *The Marriage of Heaven and Hell*.
Foulkes S. and Anthony E. (1957) *Group Psychotherapy—The Psycho-Analytic Approach*. Harmondsworth: Penguin.

Friedman M. (1985) *The Healing Dialogue*. New York: Jason Aronson, p. 97.
Jung C. (1928) *Contributions to Analytical Psychology*. Trans. H. and C. Baynes. London: Kegan Paul, Trench, Trubner, p. 116
Lewin K. (1936) *Principles of Topological Psychology*. New York: McGraw-Hill.
Perls F., Hefferline R. and Goodman P. (1951) *Gestalt Therapy*, Vol. 2. New York: Julian Press.
Stern D. (1985) *The Interpersonal World of the Infant*. New York: Basic Books.
Tobin S. (1990) Self-psychology as a bridge between existential–humanistic psychology and psychoanalysis. *Journal of Humanistic Psychology* **30**(1): 16.

Chapter 8

Wednesday morning: Dialogue

Jan writes: It is very exciting to me that you have spent a session focussing on this therapeutic style. Provided all the people concerned agree to the method, I see it as the most fruitful one for most verbal tasks within all systems, from international relations, to running organisations, to one-on-one therapy. That is a big generalisation, and I'm sticking with it.

Dialogue, which in origin means no more than talking through, must have been the commonest use of leisure time for humans, since they had language enough to manage it. Berne (1964) describes some of this conversation as pastimes. In ordinary usage are pegorative terms like chat and gossip. What is less acknowledged is that alongside these desultory or pernicious exercises of speech, go many important social tasks. One is making sense of events. Another, related, is the common agreement of meaning. A third is social, the digestion of experience, in which each speaker is guided by his or her own judgement, and argues or agrees facts and opinion and feeling until whatever is being talked of loses interest and is left behind. Such conversation is probably repetitive and can be longwinded. It is common for educated people to mock it where they overhear it happening among people who set less value than they do on wit and cleverness. Television, radio, books and newspapers, accustom many of us to passive taking in of the thoughts of others. So we need to learn the careful skill of the sort of truth-seeking dialogue which is the subject of this session reported by Sohan.

Sohan's account

Once more we met in the library, as the grass seemed still damp after the rain of the night time. There was much yawning, and most interesting talk of ways of remembering dreams. This I will attempt, as I dream too often only of that journey from my village on which my dear mother passed away and I with my father had to make a burial for her in ground too hard to dig well.

Sappho reported that she was very happy, but that she had no dreams to tell this morning. Pierre seemed still pale, and said that he had not slept well. Annie said to him in joke, "You must be in love." Quite without smiles he said yes, and I was most curious to know with whom that might be. But seeing Grace colour up, I stayed quiet, as did we all.

Perhaps fifteen minutes passed in this interesting conversation, in which I took my part. I was surprised when Chuck asked whether we might start. For me we had started. But I regret that I had not noticed the absence of Manfred, who by chance came in at this moment. After he had sat and there was quiet, Birde asked how he was. A bruise showed beside his left eye, and I fear that it will spread to be a proper black eye. He said it did not hurt.

Annie shifted from side to side as she often does before speaking, then asked if we were grown-up enough to be anarchists. I did not know I was one, so I was full of interest for this subject. She explained that the Gestalt responsibility seemed to make us all try to be all things at all times, making us too responsible in all circumstances. She argued that just as we allowed without difficulty that Manfred should organise the catering rota, so might other persons in turn perhaps be the group leader. Many people laughed, and mention was made of re-inventing the wheel, to which Grace replied that wheels were objects of great usefulness.

With some puzzlement we recalled our plan the first night of having rotating leadership, and the way we in part forgot that, and yet had given several people special leadership powers at different meetings. Annie pointed out that we had not distinguished between a tuition role, to teach our different—I think she said craft—skills, and a management role. Manfred told of a theory called Open Systems (Von Bertalanffy 1968), and of Owen's theory, which developed from this work, and that of Rice and Miller of management as a service task to the group (Owen 1978). So far as I understand, this means that the task of the manager is to manage the boundaries of the group, to allow in and out what should be let in and out, also to stop invasion, and so leave freedom for other group members to pursue their tasks in peace.

This conversation was a great clarifier to my mind. I see that in my art groups at the hospital I wish first to be teacher, to teach the simple skill of using art materials without fear and expectation. After that, much of my work is to see that paint and paper and clay and suitable new members are brought into the group, and to help patients arrange counselling meetings or art displays in their wards, which I now see are the crossings of the boundaries of the art group, back into the hospital. Just as a cell in an organism, the group takes in from the rest of the organisation, and feeds back to it.

It is all too easy to be so fascinated with the happenings inside the group, that the background on which it is figure becomes obscured. (I speak Gestalt!)

Birde reminded people of our agreement about disclosures. At this there was suddenly silence. I saw many staring at the floor and quite different in manner from some moments before, when all was lightness and discussion and joking.

Orminda said that a dream was all she had to disclose. I put down here her words from the tape.

"Do you know when a dream seems a big dream? This one was in colour, I think, and I woke from it tantalised, on the edge of understanding something that is still not there. Or maybe I knew it in the dream, the way Annie knew something extraordinary in that vision of hers. Only she has the head for making sense, and I'm as tongue-tied as the day I was born. What I remember was being in an opera, or else watching it, or both. Four characters were on the front of stage, with the chorus up at the back. Verdi's Don Carlos comes to my mind now I'm telling it, for the quality of the music. There were three male singers and one woman, and the music was all one indivisible great river, out of which came sailing now one wonderful voice and song, now another, each different, but each generated by the one before, leading ineluctably to the one coming after, supported, changed, made greater by the orchestra and the harmonies and antiphonies of the chorus. Now I get the feeling some of the group were the singers."

When people questioned her, she was not clear about which

members might have been represented in her dream, but said that the important element for her was the memory of the music, which she explained made for her an illustration of the background and figure of Gestalt.

"None of the characters had a story and feelings and need except in relation to the others," she told us. "I never before had such a sense of the total bloody myth of the individual. *The self is forged in interaction*" (Sullivan 1953).

Annie said, "Only connect," and many people nodded or smiled. I felt ashamed to ask why, so said nothing. I notice to myself that I do this I think more than is good for me.

I hope I show clearly here the wonderful colour and richness of Orminda's memory of her dream, told in her soft Irish voice with such fluency and passion. The dream, I see now, set the feeling of the morning session. And as I write that I slip into supposing the possibility that the feeling of the group produced in her the dream. Like the chorus of her opera, she sang a theme back to us to make it more clear. These are strange inspired imaginings, which I generally associate more with painting than with words. But painting is my job.

It was decided that Grace should work a little with Orminda, in what was termed the dialogue manner. Grace told very clearly how the dialogue is to do with allowing into your mind the other person, and then noticing what truly happens to you, and telling that back. Then she looked at Orminda and was quiet, before saying, "I am almost hearing your opera still, with that excitement of recognising wonderful quality of sound, of composition, of interaction." Orminda smiled and said yes, and then put out her hand and took Grace's for a moment.

"I am upset that you hold hands," said Pierre. "I tell my true response, which makes me ashamed and must be said. I agitate myself in seeing this." Truly I was a little annoyed that he broke the quiet moment with his words.

"Notice what you want to do, Pierre," said Birde. Grace looked across at her and said, "I felt alarm when you spoke. And now a tenderness, all coloured by the opera. Now we are singing an aria for one man and three women. The word rival is in my awareness. Birde, I am frightened as I intrude. And I want you to admit *your* experience, rather than telling Pierre what to do."

Birde blushed very much and I think also her eyes seemed wet, though she looked downwards and I could not be sure of this. Then she replied, "I would like to touch Pierre." He put his head in his hands and stared down also. The moment was extremely tense. Birde looked over at Grace and nodded and said, "Until this moment I had not understood that I wanted to touch Pierre. I was the so-called helpful therapist, thinking of his projections, not of mine. Now I understand better this phenomenology. We co-create, and in my work so often I deny this."

"All about touch. It is all about touch," said Sappho, stretching her arms back in what I perceived as a sexual manner. With difficulty I add, to give respect to our law of disclosure, that I have many sexual longings myself. It is now four days since I was with my wife. Sappho sits often in such a manner that it is difficult not to gaze on her thighs, and she moves also like a dancer, to show her breasts and the curve of her neck and shoulders. But I feel my longings not towards her, though she arouses me, but towards Orminda. This is most curious, as Orminda I must say wears most ugly sandals and has freckled skin. This afternoon perhaps I tell this yearning I have, as I believe strongly as Pierre tells us that the secrets are a poison to the group. But I feel the blood drain from my skin as I imagine doing so. I have interrupted the narrative, which I now resume.

At about this time Chuck put out his hand and took Sappho's, and she sighed and leant against him, with much evidence of enjoying the contact. Orminda said that she had the same feeling as in her dream, that the scene was ending, the lights were going down, but the plot was more complicated at this moment, not more resolved.

Grace seemed to be so present, the picture comes to my mind that she was levitating. Please understand that this was not so, but merely an image that comes to my mind. She said the word "Richness", and then, "Anguish".

"Rich as syllabub, deep as the Liffey. Not so much anguished," Orminda replied. I felt a body change in myself, a relief. Pierre looked up at Grace, and around at the rest of us, and said, "For me, the word is anguish. Like Orminda, each of us carries a personal opera, which must affect the opera we make together here. I need to speak of my contempt, which I would—what was this word from last night?—which I would exorcise. Look for the polarities, says Grace, says Birde." I think he was most sensitive to include Birde's name just here. "For me the polarity of contempt is charity. Never have I had enough of this. Always have I suffered arrogance."

"There is some response in my arms, in my veins, I think," said Grace. "I may be feeling the charity you are not finding. And the image comes to me of you scourging yourself in public." He listened with his mouth drawn down, in that way which looks so severe, but which I now recognise as concentration. I think to myself that his patients might at times feel frightened of him as I do.

"Yes," he said, "The public scourging. I began it but I scorn it. On that I spit." Chuck and Sappho laughed, and Chuck moved so that he was in contact with Manfred as well as Sappho. Manfred laughed too, and I think all smiled, especially when Pierre himself, instead of becoming angry as I had feared, smiled at his own complicated contempt of his contempt.

Then he told of his clinically depressed wife. From the hospital I know some such cases, of people telling such lies, being so destructive of their families. "Ideas of reference" I remember my dear friend Dr Anscombe calling this. Pierre's wife for several years believed their son's school was trying to turn the child against her, then that Pierre had stolen an inheritance. She wrote to colleagues and newspapers and made much trouble, even coming to his consulting rooms and threatening suicide many times. Now she is in a hospital, and his son is brought up by his cousin and mother for the moment.

Grace said, "And you tell that story now, so it becomes part of this opera. Now I hear the word anguish in my mind again. I remember how easy it is for me to play the toughy. I do it by joking."

"And I by the sneering," said Pierre. "But now I am troubled. In this group, this river of sound, this Liffey Orminda speaks of and that I have never seen, starts again. I had forgotten anguish and longing, the nostalgia for—*la jouissance*."

"Joy," said Orminda. But he repeated the French word.

"La jouissance" said Annie softly, adding that she did not know the word.

Orminda said that all this conversation had for her seemed a continuation of the opera of her dream, and that she had heard the rhythms and the music of what was said, in a way that had never happened for her before.

"The voices came out of the group. The group generated the voices," she said, and then added that she was frightened of interrupting what was happening by trying to analyse it. I had a feeling of roundedness in what each had been saying, and wished very much that I had ever seen an opera, so I could have more sense of her vision. We stopped at about this time to take coffee and so on, and met again by the pond in a few minutes, as the sun was now as hot as at any time in the week.

Manfred was carrying a book, from which he read aloud, but without explanation, as soon as everyone had arranged themselves in or out of the shade of the walnut tree:

"...if you and I were clever savants, and the examination of the content of our hearts was a thing of the past ... we'd meet, as sophists do, with great clashing of argument on argument. But as it is, since we're amateurs, our first concern will be to compare our thoughts, to see what they are, whether they are consistent or quite opposite."

Having our attention, he then told us that he was reading the words of the philosopher Plato, put in the mouth of Socrates in a book called *The Theaetetus*. He told us that Plato was giving a description of the dialogue method, which Manfred said was becoming the most respected way of work in many schools of psychotherapy. He then read a little more:

"There's plenty of time. We don't need to be impatient. What we're really looking at is ourselves, to see what these phantoms are that lurk within us."

I felt great shame, that I had not well understood the several references to the dialogue method made by Grace and Annie. Luckily I was not alone in my ignorance, and the fearlessness of others in exposing themselves encouraged me to ask many questions and make a good understanding. With the help of the tape I write some of that here.

Grace was indeed graceful this morning, and seemed very animated to find that Plato described dialogue in many ways as she would. She spoke eagerly:

"I think of Plato's dialogues as intellectual, as about abstractions. But here he is acknowledging the personal, the phenomenological. What he calls the phantoms that lurk within are to me all the responses your presence and actions generate in me. Just now I am shifting your habit of quotation from my prejudice that it is a grey, avoidant, self-conquering habit. Now I feel the depth of your letting other thinkers into this conversation. What I respond to you has to be a product of this totality Annie spoke of, the totality of all my own experience, and all that is informed and informing, in every cell of my body. I see you now with all these associations to the great thinkers and perceivers, and notice the envy that was under my impatience with you before." She spoke with such warmth that I greatly wished Manfred to be as generous to her. But he simply nodded. I was most grateful to hear Chuck speak next:

"Just let me get this straight. You said dialogue was talking through, right? Now the bit that seems to have lit up Grace from that quotation is what I guess she'd call the phenomenological, the catching hold of the subjective phenomena of response, and reporting them to the first speaker?" When she agreed he went on, "So dialogue is a kind of honesty exercise, being on the level, telling back what really happens for me when, say when Manfred pisses off in group time. Knocking him down was acting out. It wasn't dialogue. If I'd told you, or told the others, since you weren't there, that I was mad... But I did. Yeah, but I left out the internal phenomena. I got a little teleological at that point, I remember."

"Dialogue is existential. It is of the moment," said Grace. Chuck looked straight at Manfred and said:

"OK. The now from me to you is shame, a lot of that still. Really wanting to abase myself, in a way that takes my memory back to the way I got pushed around when I was a kid. And the way I pushed my sister around. And coming back from that dive down my past, seeing you nod and look back, really look at me now, I get what I'd call a brotherly feeling, though I haven't a brother." The two men stood and embraced, there on the grass, and my heart was very full to see such warmth expressed in this country, as I remember it from mine.

When they sat down, Birde spoke slowly, "Now I see this equality between the dialogue speakers, each to be so open. I love this. Yet I think, how can I be thus with certain patients? How to tell my boredom with one, or my disapproval at the drinking habits of another?"

"My sense of the context helps me," Grace replied. "I feel my disapproval, say. And I know that I am therapist in this conversation, and that my client probably gives more power to what I say than someone else might. So my disapproval is already qualified inside me before I speak. I respond to my idea of over-drinking, and at the same time to my memory of some of the underlying context in which that client drinks, and to my knowledge of her likely response to direct disapproval." Birde sighed and said that she understood Grace very well, and saw how her own technique must improve. Annie said that she saw how her whole spirit must improve. Then she added:

"I am thinking of another place where the open, the on-the-level, horizontal dialogue might not be therapeutically useful. For instance, one of my patients said as she was leaving the house, 'I am so glad that you have lots of young children.' Now I have not. But my training led me to smile and say nothing, and then to direct her attention to this statement at the beginning of the next session. She had seen several different coloured anoraks of mine hanging on pegs in the hall, and, I suppose from her needs to mother and be mothered, managed to ignore the length of the sleeves, and see them as children's coats. Now I suspect she learned more from persisting in her folly and becoming wise for herself, than if I had butted in straight away with an impulsive assertion of the true position."

"I notice you look across at me," said Grace, "and feel a bit of alarm, that I am taking on the role of dialogue expert. I imagine a question in you, which you know how to answer." Their eyes met and then Annie laughed and nodded, and said:

"My training is as much part of me as my impulse to correct an error. That's the background from which I acted, instead of just responding to impulse. So I was dialogic, in a way."

"When you two giggled just now," said Orminda to Grace and Annie, "I imagined that as one of those rare I–Thou moments of intense meeting Buber (1974) talks about. They've been thick as fleas in this group this morning."

"There was a definite jolt in my insides," said Grace, "somewhere round that chakra in the belly. A sort of triumph in meeting. For me."

"Yes," said Annie, "The creation of the between, the we. Friedman (1985) calls it something like that."

"Also between Chuck and myself," said Manfred, "I have experienced strongly this essential condition of growth, this momentary and overwhelming healthy confluence. Like the orgasm, it is of short duration but great significance." There was some silence after this. I have noticed this often after Manfred speaks (De Mare 1975). In my humble opinion, it is difficult for him to connect to the future, to the next person, so that the dialogue is a ball thrown from one and lightly caught by another. His strength is to connect from the past. He holds the ball, failing even to make eye contact with others when he speaks. I regret that I did not contribute this idea to the discussion. But at the time I was very excited at this recognition of the beautiful moments I have sometimes known, when a patient and I seem to meet, perhaps without words, but in a way that is most enriching to me.

"I have noticed that you don't ask many questions in this dialogue mode," said Sappho to Grace. "That means you show yourself, more than try to control the interlocutor. I want you to tell some more of the technique of dialogue. Speak about that intervention category some Gestaltist made up, that you were talking about at supper last night."

"You mean John Frew (1992)? He has this lovely simple idea of three categories of intervention. He's talking about group leaders, but for me it applies anywhere, and from anyone to anyone. I either impose on, or compete with or confirm you in whatever I do or say to you. Imposing is getting you to do things because I figure they're a good idea, or getting you to see my point of view or understand yourself within my frame of reference or whatever. Contesting is often there in certain styles of phenomenological dialogue. If Annie had said to her patient something like, 'You imagine me with lots of children, and like me the more for that. And now I feel anxious that you may like me less, because I only have two adolescents,' that would have been a contesting statement. Her reality would have been put, albeit gently, in contest against the other person's."

"And the confirming one," said Birde, her voice seeming to take up from Grace's so naturally that I remembered the dream of the opera, "might be just the reflection, 'Many young children is a picture of joyfulness to you'. But only if I reflected accurately, of course. And perhaps that lady received Annie's return to the subject the next week as confirming. A confirming imposition."

"You got it," said Grace. "There's what I intend, and there's what you hear, and they can be poles apart. But it comes to me now, that the I–Thou probably only happens when there's an underlying confirmatory stance in both people, for that moment at least."

"I am thinking," said Pierre, "that my analyst makes only confirmations to me. No question ever, no contest, no imposition. And each statement if ever she speaks, so centrally meeting the anguish of what I mean but am in the dark to see or express."

"Either that, or you're locked in a God-awful dependency," said Grace. Pierre looked up at her sharply, and she added, "I don't know why I said that." He shrugged, and there was silence.

I heard myself say, "The dialogue stopped."

"Yes," said Annie. "In the silence I remembered Manfred's quotation. Plato said something about having plenty of time, and no need to be impatient. Talking through takes so much time. I recognise how often I do that cut-off that Grace and Pierre seem to have done now."

"For this moment they are the protagonists, and we are the Greek chorus," said Orminda. "Do you hear how we state the present, then comment, expand it? We are the environment of their sub-group."

"I prefer the idea of Greek chorus. These Gestalt words are unspeakable (Cohn 1970)," said Annie. "I'm not an environment." She looked at Pierre, then longer at Grace, and added quietly, "I feel anguish, this word that has been said, between you. And I want a happy ending."

"Not today, Napoleon," said Grace.

Annie said, "Excuse me," and began searching in a shabby large book she had on the grass beside her. She read out, "Jung says, '...*a neurosis is more a psychosocial phenomenon than an illness in the strict sense. It forces us to extend the term illness beyond the idea of an individual body whose functions are disturbed, and to look upon the neurotic person as a sick system of social relationships.*' And there's another bit, a very Gestalt bit, it's here on page 224: '*Wholeness is the result of an intrapsychic process which depends essentially on the relation of one individual to another.*' Just seeing you two now, I remembered those words."

"Yes, it is I who am the neurotic person," said Pierre. "I make around me the sick system of relationships. And in this web I trap Grace now. She speaks within my intrapsychic dialogue just now. She speaks from my contempt, my need to diminish. She is trapped in a projective identification."

"My mood has changed so completely," said Grace. "I was on top of the world. Then suddenly I sniped at Pierre like that, thoughtlessly. It's somehow like Chuck and Manfred last night. Wholeness." She put her hand over her heart and sighed, "Where shall I get it?"

"I hope from everyone," said Orminda.

"You know," said Chuck, "I don't know if anyone's come up with categories of dialogue, but I just kind of thought some up. That getting trapped into someone else's patterns like Pierre says Grace did just now: you could call that intrapsychic dialogue, like he did. Or marionette dialogue. One pulls the strings and the other acts powerless. There's a hell of a lot of conversation like that in the world. In my language, it involves projective identification. I guess in Gestalt you'd explain it as projection by one, and introjection by the other. And it has no place in therapy.

Then I was thinking how tired I can be when I've been working with some manic or schizophrenic patients. We have conversations in which I do know that honesty is my only protection. God, psychotic people have a nose for what's phoney. But I'm like that civil servant guy, I'm economical with the truth. I keep a hold of the field we are both operating in, and speak from that. So someone tells me he's planning on leaving the hospital, or starting a business from inside the ward, or some damn thing. And I'll probably say a straight imposition, like, 'I really don't want you to do that, Fred. I'm thinking of how you want to lead a normal life and be free of hospital routines, and I don't want you to get excited at the moment, or you'll be back on heavier medication.' That kind of thing works. It's apparently very open. But I'm holding on for all I'm worth to my good feelings for that patient as I speak. I'm looking at their world and just dropping in a little of my doctor-world. It works, nine times out of ten. And people say I'm so frank and easy and all. But I'm battening down a right power-punch of irritation or worry, half the time. I'd call that a therapeutic dialogue, not a free one.

Now with some patients I do get to what I'm calling a free dialogue. Maybe more than with a lot of my family or friends."

Grace was listening intently, nodding very much. Now she took up what he was saying, in the way that again makes me think of the singing voices that continue from one to another: "I love that. You've come up with such clear categories. Using Gestalt words to describe the same thing, I suppose the joining in someone else's patterned dialogue, making the responses they expect rather than what are more centrally mine, could be called confluent dialogue. Then that pretty full, but still careful therapeutic style reminds me of what Gordon Wheeler describes as being the environment for the other. I could shorthand to a jargon phrase for us, Environment Dialogue. But this last you were just coming to—I suppose Contact Dialogue would be an orthodox description. But God, that word is limited. To me it's not big enough to describe the penetration, the receptivity, the sense of bodily change, that happens at those unlooked for moments of what seems total mutuality and understanding."

"With these words you make love to Chuck, I think," said Pierre. Grace shook her head. Then Manfred cut in:

"So this group is a co-operative system now. It demonstrates the dialogue of which we speak."

I ventured to express a muddled idea of mine, that perhaps we could miss beats and then come in the right rhythm, when the dialogue is flowing deep as Orminda's Irish river. Even this seemed understood by all. I know I had spoken as I did, partly in response to Manfred, who might at other times have seemed to cut across the conversation of others. Now we expanded, I think, to allow in his more abstract thought.

Jan's comment

The Perls–Simkin polarity

By now you are around the middle of this group's life. More and more self-revelation, in recounting and in action, has happened. Members' empathic abilities are in use. In Gestalt terms, you are in the Contact phase. In this phase, the subject is less the figure than the activity that is engaged in: I am what I do.

Orminda dreams you into being an opera. That is one of the group forms of art that most obviously generates and allows emotionality and value. What strikes her more is unity of expression, synchronicity of perception. Each action or feeling within the group is now perceived as belonging to all. But of course you are still different characters; you still have your own identities.

All this is about the sense of the group as an entity. It is about belonging, awarely.

That is a wonderful image, of you as something as powerful and moving as an opera. Like many operas, you have recurrent themes. Leadership versus anarchy is still spoken of. Self-disclosure continues, in ways that seem to make people ever more acceptant of themselves and each other. The social climate is that of a learning group, in what Marton and Saljo (1976) call deep-level processing. Bales' (1951) *phase hypothesis, of nesting* of task activities, and a consequent building of tension which is expressed in emotional release, is again discernible. It echoes the Gestalt notion of certain polarities. Where Gestalt differs from the equilibrium theorists is in its attention to growth and change, rather than what is after all a myth of homeostasis.

Sexual feeling is beginning to emerge with all the power, and in Pierre's word, anguish, that are familiar in many operas. I acknowledge anxiety, as I wonder whether it will stay at this somewhat camouflaged level, or erupt among you with the pain that is likely for such people as you are.

I move to the calmer ground of talking, as I had promised, of dialogue and Gestalt. Fritz Perls is said to have been a brilliant diagnostician. He practised this skill at all opportunities, guessing and checking on the lives of people in restaurants and in the street, as well as in therapeutic meetings. In his later years he demonstrated the range of experimental techniques of Gestalt, which can be brilliant, showy, fast and effective, and thus gratifying to his personality. These often brief public interventions came from this background of huge diagnostic skill and clinical experience. His style has often been copied, without the accompanying experience.

Laura Perls, Jim Simkin, Erving and Miriam Polster and others who attended Perls' early seminars in New York, represent a far more dialogic tradition. Perhaps because he wrote less, or had a less exciting technique, Jim Simkin's persistence with a dialogic interpretation of Gestalt therapeutic method has remained less known. I know Grace has attended some of Gary Yontef's events, and so has probably influenced this session into being an example of dialogue at the same time as a description of it. Latterly, Gary has done as much as anyone to remind us of the particular Gestalt experiment of dialogue itself. He points out that Jim Simkin insisted publicly on the I and Thou, here and now character of Gestalt. In

Gary's view, Gestalt dialogue has been developed more fully by later practitioners, of whom he is clearly one of the most informed models.

Orminda's and Chuck's categorisation into intrapsychic, therapeutic, and full dialogue, re-named by Grace Confluent, Environment and Contact Dialogue, clarified a lot for me. It made me see that I would not call what you name Confluent Dialogue as dialogue at all, though I admire your pointing up this therapeutic and social bear trap. You are starting in on that honing of theory I hoped for when I set up our residential in the first place. Your ideas come from the particular, from the moment, from the dialogue itself, and are the more comprehensible as well as the sounder for that.

That has me dreaming of how a dialogic mind-set on all sides might transform any group or system, to allow out more of the meaning and value of its members. Generations of education are needed to make any such dream capable of enactment. So, vite, vite, there is not a moment to lose.

References

Bales R. (1951) *Interaction Process Analysis: A Method for the Study of Small Groups*. Cambridge: Addison-Wesley.

Berne E. (1964) *Games People Play*. New York: Grove Press.

Buber M. (1974) Dialogue. In: *Between Man and Man*. London: Kegan Paul.

Cohn R. (1970) Therapy in groups. In: J. Fagan and I. L. Shepherd (Eds), *Gestalt Therapy Now*. New York: Harper Colophon, pp. 137–138.

De Mare P. (1975). In: L. Kreeger (Ed.), *The Large Group*. London: Maresfield Reprints, p. 27.
> "Dr de Mare expounded his distinction between the hierarchical leader, where interventions bring communication to a full stop, and the spokesman of leading ideas, who appears now from one part of the group, now another."

Frew J. (1992) The art of intervention in Gestalt group psychotherapy. Presentation at Gestalt Journal Conference, Boston.

Friedman M. (1985) *The Healing Dialogue*. New York: Jason Aronson.

Hycner R.H. (1991) *Between Person and Person: Towards a Dialogical Psychotherapy*. Highland, New York: Gestalt Journal Press.

Jung (1954) The practice of psychotherapy. In: *Collected Works*, Vol. 16, Trans. R. Hull. New York: Pantheon, pp. 178 and 224.

Langs R. (1982) *The Psychotherapeutic Conspiracy*. New York: Aronson.
Marton F. and Saljo R. (1976) On qualitative differences in learning: 1 and 2, *British Journal of Educational Psychology* 46: 1 and 2.
Owen T. (1978) *Making Organisations Work*. Leiden: Martin Nijhoff.
Plato. *Theaetetus*, Trans. R. Waterfield. Harmondsworth: Penguin, 1987, p. 36.
Simkin J. and Yontef G. (1984) Gestalt therapy. In: R. Corsini (Ed.), *Current Psychotherapies*. Ithasca, Ill.: Peacock.
Smith D (1991) *Hidden Conversations. An Introduction to Communicative Psychoanalysis*. London: Routledge.
Sullivan H.S. (1953) *The Interpersonal Theory of Psychiatry*. New York: W.W. Norton.
Von Bertalanffy L. (1968) General Systems Theory. In: W. Buckley (Ed.) *Modern Systems Research for the Behavioral Scientist*. Chicago: Aldine.
Yontef G. (1981) Mediocrity and Excellence: an Identity Crisis in Gestalt Therapy. ERIC/CAPS, University of Michigan, Ed. 214,062.

Chapter 9

Wednesday afternoon: Pairing

Jan writes: The pair, seen by some theorists as the basis of all social organisation (Simmel 1950), is salient this afternoon. Hints and more than hints have been shown to us from the first session. Now we have most of the orchestra take up the theme, at times with almost overwhelmed urgency. The pair seems so figural, that it is evoked in its most consummate form, the sexual. Once more, there is confusion for maybe all of you, about whether you have just happened to coincide in experiencing private feelings, whether you are the victims of the gods, of some collective force which clouds your judgement, or whether what is experienced as sexually urgent is a metaphor for other transactions.

What I need, ashamedly, to confess, is that by Wednesday I was stuck in Salonika, and had found out how to go by train and boat to England, a journey which would only get me to you by Thursday evening. Then, quite by chance at a bus station, I met a woman I had known many years ago. We told each other that the strike would soon be over, and that she would be free to go by air to Italy, and me to England, and thus we argued ourselves into spending the evening together. I too was enmeshed in a pair whose significance was not very clear to me. Jung (1959) might smile at this confession of synchronicity. That I got food-poisoning later that evening was a twist to the story, and the only part I let you know at the time.

Birde's account

Much is different since last I sat to write the happenings in one of our group meetings. To think of that first evening is to look back to childhood hopes, from sad middle age.

They do not need me, this group. Many can do, and do better, what I can. So, by writing this record, I behave again like the spinster aunt, making preserves in the kitchen while the young ones play.

The theme of the two hours was what Manfred calls sub-groups of two. It is true to say that we did not ever move completely from our first task of the session, our disclosures. This I began, with an effort of courage, to tell how touched I had been that Chuck held my hands when we went swimming in the deep pool that Sappho had found at one bend of the brook, under the trees. I cannot swim, and wanted so much to try once more.

Chuck made all safe with his large steady hands and his warm eyes. With his help I let go and felt my legs free in the water, felt it float me upwards. What was to disclose was my excitement that I could swim, and more, the ridiculous burst of love feelings I had to Chuck. I remember saying that because he made me special in the group, I had become a different person. As he smiled across at me, I let myself say all: the erotic feelings that he had seen me naked; the sudden dream that he and I should do some workshops together this winter, which I could arrange in my country.

He said he would like to work with me. All were quiet and intent since I began, and soon I understood that all minds, or many, worked the same ways.

Grace at this time said to Chuck that she doubted if I wanted him to respond warmly only to the idea of workshops. She turned her head to look full at Pierre and added, "A workshop sounds like what you call a work group. Don't you think Birde was more interested in the affect group (Bion 1961)?"

"Please ask Birde this," said Pierre, with his most Parisian shrug. Annie commented on the pang she felt, like something cold through her stomach, when Pierre responded in this way to Grace.

"What the hell are you two up to?" she asked Pierre and Grace, then added, "Now I'm adopting Chuck's therapeutic style of speech. You're a very powerful group member, Chuck."

"Well I don't feel it," he answered. I have it clear on the tape.

"I feel pretty well invisible and inaudible most of the time, until I put my foot in it." Sohan said that he wished to know more of Annie's remarks to Grace and Pierre.

"Yesterday Grace snubbed Pierre, right out of the blue. And regularly, you smack her down when she says something to draw you in."

"To draw him into the pair," I added. "I have noticed that he rebels when Grace speaks a little privately to him, he resists very much. Ah, there is his word, resist! Pierre too is powerful, or at least, I give him great power here."

"So we give power to the men," said Annie, and we exchanged glances and I felt a warmth to her which was most comforting. It was again like this dream of the morning, the opera, in which different voices expand one theme without disputes. "I give power to you too, Birde," she added. "For this is a Gestalt phrase that you use often. I let you influence me. That is more accurate than the usual speech forms."

"You know what I think?" said Chuck suddenly, "I think Jan is having a hectic love affair somewhere, and is spending the whole of this week in bed with a woman." Grace did her best to imitate Pierre's manner, and said to Chuck:

"Would you care to associate to the projective element in that statement?" Chuck blushed crimson, and Grace added, "Thank you, doctor. I see that you are taking me seriously." She spoke in a joking tone. But from then all seemed serious and difficult between us, as I had felt it earlier when I hinted my feelings for Chuck. I understand from the tape how quickly I was set aside after I had spoken, and that makes me more forgiving of my childish feelings which came up at times in the session.

Annie said, after swallowing once or twice, "Since my divorce I have felt so wary of male contact. But Chuck reminds me of how good it is to smell a man's sweat. I imagine being held in dependable arms, being at peace." She looked across at Chuck as she spoke, and I am absolutely sure that all this was a statement to him. I tell in parenthesis that I had no sense of rivalry with me, but more of our being caught in the same boat, the same yearning. However, Manfred responded, also after throat-clearings.

"Of course there is inevitability in experiencing such sexual needs, when thrown together in a system of this kind. Structure affects content and process. I remember the words of Patrick de

Mare (1975). Yet it is with great turmoil that I admit that last night, Annie, I had a dream of being in a bed with you. I was knowing that soon we would make love with great success." He looked down and put his hand across his eyes, looking far from successful.

"Thank you, I am very flattered," said Annie quietly, adding, "I imagine that it must be difficult for you to forgive these transferential inevitabilities, when your wife and marriage are so important to you?" He nodded, staccato, without looking up. It seemed a dialogue moment, even though anyone glancing at the scene would have thought him quite out of contact. I felt a sadness for him, for my guess is that the marriage is not perhaps as wonderful as he needs to believe it. Annie's and my eyes met, and I know we shared the same guess, and the same feeling. I tried to convey that I knew she had thought of Chuck, not Manfred, when she spoke, and that I had great admiration for her not being so fully disclosing as Pierre likes us to be.

Manfred will leave tomorrow. Let him take his belief system with him, since there is not time to let him grow a new one. Now as I write an insight comes to me, and I am happy. I was piqued that in this group, as in all places, there is no male who wishes to pair with me. But I have a strong partner in Annie. So strange that I disliked her so greatly the first night. And now, without our having a great fight or drama, she is my friend. She is the one I could work with, for I see that our training is so different, and also our personalities, but still we have the same way of looking at the depth of the world. Chuck has warmth to patients; but I too have that. He has a very reassuring and earthy response, which I can copy, without having to import him to supply it. Good!

Like a cat who sits down in the midst of a fight, to lick its leg, I think in telling this aside I was partly making a displacement activity too. The tension in our circle was very high. Sappho and Orminda both lay on their stomachs and tore up the drying grass round them, with the sound of sheep grazing. Sappho said defiantly, "Chuck and I make a pair. Look around the group! We are the nearest in age."

"This is an allegation," said Pierre. "Orminda also is in your age bracket, if this is the ridiculous way you have to choose."

"The disclosure is the phenomenology, the telling of your experi-

Pairing

ence in the moment," Grace added. "*All knowledge takes its place within the horizons opened up by perception* (Merleau-Ponty 1962)."

"You cook your own saucepans. I cook mine," said Sappho, sounding nine years old.

"Quite right," said Grace. "I'm still aware of not answering Annie when she asked what was going on between me and Pierre. Well, I can't speak for him. But I have a feeling that is an echo of what Sappho has just said. To me, Pierre and I are a pair. Other people have said that, I know. But I feel it." She looked as if she spoke with great effort, to seem light.

"Only theory can help us here," said Pierre, quite pale. Several of us smiled at the desperate tone he used, to make such an intellectual remark. "It is a commonplace to sexualise, to cathect in this way. But it is quite a transient emotion, only of this place."

"Of course," said Manfred in agreement. "Without any doubt you two have become a pair in this group. Pierre represents the knowledge of unconscious process, and Grace the knowledge of Gestalt. They are a monarchic pair. So comes to them the romantic idea that the monarchs are also the passionate lovers. But this is not a systemic requirement. It is perhaps a biological requirement, which I alone am in an easy position to fulfil soon."

"I am suffering," said Grace. "I have some of what I think Birde and Annie have hinted at: a vulnerable, atavistic, yearning, waiting to be swept on to the white charger and carried securely off, feeling. Yes, I run workshops on fairy stories, to point up how to resist all this male-oriented conditioning. But here I go. I feel about sixteen, and gauche with it." She raised her head to look at Pierre, who did not return the glance. Instead he said, "Now I feel the *maudissement*, the curse of this disclosure I propose, and which I have not made. So there is my first disclosure."

"Chuck said he felt invisible here," said Sappho, interrupting Pierre in the sudden way I have come to expect from her. "You're trying to do the same to me. Nobody has answered me about me and Chuck." There was a moment of silence. She had interrupted Pierre at what felt a crucial moment, and I think we waited for him to discipline her. But he did not.

"Yes, I fear many things stay unsaid," said Sohan nervously, and went on, "These feelings some people speak of, I too have with great intensity, and my thoughts are quite full of Orminda, but of course I assure you with no wish for imposition. Only I confess this."

His timing was terrible. "Shut up!" said Sappho to him, and Annie interrupted, "Now do you all know why I said we needed a chairperson? I'm taking the role, if everyone agrees."

"You do not listen to me!" Sappho said, very loud. Two nuns were walking not far away, and I was anxious they did not gain a bad impression of our group. In spite of Sappho's interruptions, we quickly agreed that Annie was chairperson for the rest of the session. She became quite different in this role, almost brisk, as she asked that people should only speak if they had raised their hand and had her permission. Sappho shrieked angrily at this, but Chuck turned on her, remembering almost too late to raise his hand before doing so, and spoke to her quite severely. I thought to myself that perhaps the little sister he said he had locked in a barn had been as egocentric as Sappho. He is the only one of us who can handle her in her hysterical moments.

Now suddenly all was silence again and I waited to see who would raise their hand. Poor Sohan looked troubled. Sappho had flared her nostrils and pushed her lips out. Pierre seemed to have aged twenty years, so I could imagine him a stooped and balding academic. Tears were on Grace's cheeks, and I guessed that she hoped they would dry in the sun, as she held her face up to it, rather than using a handkerchief. Orminda had twisted her hair into a rope round her hand, and seemed to be pulling steadily at it. Manfred looked at her with honest tenderness. He seemed the most open and peaceful person present. He raised his hand and said:

"The dilemma for the group is once more about multiple membership. Is it possible, is it allowed, to be half of a pair, and also to be one of this group?" His words were so near what Pierre might have said, that I marvelled again at this swallowing of each other we are all doing, mostly without open comment.

"The problem is also membership of other pairs," said Pierre bleakly.

Annie put in, "The choice before us is whether to talk at a general level, or to return to what Sohan and Sappho and Pierre had begun to say for themselves, but have not pursued."

Sappho put her hand up, though did not look for Annie's nod before saying, "You all think I am being like a child. But it is not

Pairing

easy to say these brutal things. Chuck and I are physically a magnificent pair." Pierre muttered something angry about breeding the pure race, then apologised to Annie. "Answer me, Chuck!" Sappho added.

"You're beautiful," said Chuck, "and I'll bet we could have a good time together. But Orminda, excuse me for saying this in public. I've got a lot of feeling for you." His voice conveyed the lot of feeling much more than the stilted Antipodean words. Sappho curled up in a foetal position and rolled away from him, and Grace put a hand on her back, keeping it there for a long time. Orminda bit her lips and plaited her hair the other way round her hand, seeming most embarrassed. Three men had now declared her their passion. She said faintly:

"I don't want to say anything. I just don't know what to say." She seemed overloaded, and nobody pressed her. Sohan repeated that there was no demand in what he had told her, though his looks belied these words.

"Sohan is acknowledging transience," said Manfred, in the gentle voice I remembered from that first evening, when he was designated leader. "Perhaps other people are frightened by some myth of permanence. But to belong to one pair also allows that you belong in other pairs. For the washing-up with jokes, Sohan and Chuck make a pair. For deep images, Birde and Annie." I was amazed that he could see something so subtle. "For creative dancing, Grace and Sappho are a pair. For Rogerian group ethics, Grace and Orminda. Each person here is paired at many levels with many others. Only the sexual attraction fills us with such guilt and dread, and spectres of wedding vows, no, till death do us part?" At last he used the first person plural when speaking of the group. People nodded to what he said.

The theory is easy. But here we were in the midst of the experience, and in need of such reminders, to preserve our self-esteem. I added my words, about sex only being one expression of love, and only genital expression of sex apparently being the provoker of shame. There followed a quiet conversation, in which many of us looked or said some of our love for each other. Grace quoted someone she had visited in prison, who had written a poem containing the line, "*For this moment I love you forever.*" (Daly 1973) It was of great help to us, I think.

But so much was unfinished. Manfred was so right about the

myth of permanence. The story-book part of me wanted everyone in happy little pairs, all making love without jealousy and recrimination. Privately I knew that Chuck and Orminda, and Pierre and Grace, were the only pairs who might be expressed in this way. If only they would get on with it! Of course, Sappho seemed a great difficulty in the way, as she lay there before us, rejected.

"How are you all stopping yourselves?" Annie asked, evidently thinking as I was. "Dreaming is free. You can say what or who you want now, without being enmeshed for ever."

Pierre said, "I detest to join this queue of the hungry dogs. I have shame. I am in torment, so I could wish myself with no gonads. But I think of you, Orminda, with great intensity of desire. Please understand, I have great clarity about abstinence. There is no risk I molest you. But by my rules I must tell this transferential infatuation, which is easily explained by the poignancy of your own life, and by the missing parts of my own marriage."

Sappho sat up to stare at Orminda and find her reaction. I think we were all looking the same way, and positively avoiding Grace. A pulse beat in my stomach, and I felt in shock, that Pierre's feelings were not for her after all. It was dreadful. Grace could contain this clever, passionate, petulant, indulged and deprived Frenchman. How could he pair with this vulnerable Orminda without showing his sadism, his hectoring?

But Orminda looked at him and spoke! She said that she wanted him to look after her, and added, "Abstinence is your magic talisman to avoid commitment. I don't want your abstinence like the sign of the bloody cross against me. I have no interest in your masochistic writhings in the toils of the Catholic Church. I need comfort, Pierre, and from you, as you need comfort, and from me." He looked at the ground. As in a play, I changed identification to the last speaker, and now wanted of all things that he should sleep with her. Others said encouragement of the same kind, speaking of his non-marriage, of her loneliness, of the assured confidentiality we would in any case offer.

Grace said, "Do not press him. What are you all wanting, that they are to fulfil?" Pierre said thank you to her, meeting her eyes. I admired her so much, that she did not curl up or sulk or have hysterics on her own account. She stayed with her sense of the whole group, when I was swept into awareness almost only of pairs. Sappho had looked several times at Chuck, who did not

Pairing

look back. He, like Manfred and Sohan, had much to digest at this moment.

Certainly something was strange in our intensity of interest in this pair of Pierre and Orminda. He began to speak, unsmiling, and I heard the little click sounds of his having a dry mouth. He was taking refuge in theory, his male defence. And the content of what he said interested me greatly.

"Bion's idea of the pair as flight from the group has largely been discarded or superseded in modern practice, so now we speak more of the atmosphere of expectation, the mood of expectation. Both concepts are relevant here, I think. The group attempts to use Orminda and me to give meaning to its life. We are to bring forth the Messiah." He looked not at all like God the Father, and I said so, somewhat in revenge on him for his coldness at this moment of Orminda's brave confession.

Grace interrupted, as usual to keep peace, I think, saying to Pierre, "Only you will know if you are only the instrument of all the yearning for life, for completion, that is in all of us, or whether there is also a true pairing* between you and Orminda, which you deny by reminding yourself of Bion."

"I think you over-compensate," said Pierre distantly. O my God! Why do I long for a man? They are such hateful self-centred immature little boys. Orminda shifted and spoke:

"You're talking as if Wilfred Bion was the top and bottom of the bloody wisdom of the universe, which he was not. What about Schutz? (1960) What about Affection, by which the bugger meant no more nor less than true pairing, being one of only three categories of behaviour possible in the bloody group? What about that being the health of the damned group, not its bloody sickness?" The image came to my mind of a fairy-story battle between two priests from different religions, each holding up their Holy Book and trying to explode the other with the power of it. I do not know if other people feared this power contest. In any case, we talked all as a group again, of times we had known pairs to be an avoidance of membership of the group, and times when it had been an enhancement. Annie spoke again of Plato's army of lovers,

---

* Pierre Turquet made two categories of partnership. He saw them either as dependent relationships, the needy dependent feelings attended with resentment, or as true pairs, with mutual exchange and enhancement.

each being the best of himself before his beloved, yet always being part of the whole army too.

Sohan asked in detail what Schutz meant by Affection, which helped me understand better the range of meetings of one person to one other, the Heraclitan flux of pairs that is always happening, and which is the more nourishing when admitted. Manfred instructed us all to hold hands for an experiment in perception, as he called it. To my astonishment, Pierre did not refuse, so for some moments he was holding hands with Orminda. Manfred's experiment involved noticing what he called true contact. I had to look first at Sohan on my left, then Annie on my other side. I could have contact with Chuck and Orminda opposite me. But the good feel of the two hands holding mine was in itself confluent, not contactful. It gave a sense of solidarity. Sappho for a time maintained that she could have contact with both her partners at once; then she admitted that her attention could not be fully in two directions, it could only flicker rapidly between. Manfred had offered us an experiment to make a Gestalt point!

I have read that in family therapy there are often some tricks used to change behaviour. I asked myself if part of Manfred's purpose was to bring Pierre and Orminda into the contact that Pierre forbade. There was a moment when they turned to look at each other, and I strongly believe that all the rest of us except perhaps Sappho were back into willing them to enjoy the beauty of the moment. Each so deprived in different ways; each with the horrible Catholic background that would at least help them understand each other; but there, perhaps he is not good enough for her. And yet he looked at her with such longing, as she did at him. And she was the one who broke the gaze finally.

And now I have written these judgmental and intrusive thoughts, I know that I must confess them in disclosure time next session. The temptation to cross out the words is strong. What Grace called selective authenticity (Cohn 1970) would be easier here than the truthfulness we have set ourselves. I notice how few people have circulated their reports, and ask myself if it is also because they write secrets they have difficulty to speak before us all.

Jan's comment

Birde here describes much of what makes pairing a painful subject to be avoided in many groups. Choosing is seen as sexual and as permanent, and as reflecting heavily on the worth and self-esteem of those chosen and those rejected. At this stage it is likely that Grace, Sohan, Birde, Manfred, Sappho, Chuck and Annie all have a sense of diminishment and loss. In the unusual intimacy of this life together in one house, they have, not surprisingly, done what Pierre would call sexualise their feelings to each other. Birde reminds herself that there are other kinds of pair, like that she senses with Annie. But men are a scarce resource, you seem sexually aware, and competitiveness comes easily to most of you.

Manfred described the theme of this session not as pairing, but as multiple membership. By this he meant acceptance of belonging to more than one pair or group at one time. This sounds easy enough. But a zoom function in the mind seems time and again to make membership of one group so figural that the ground of multiple membership is quite occluded. So, the pairs Bion spoke of were the pairs that seek to deny or exclude the rest. They say implicitly, "We belong in the pair therefore we do not belong in the group." This process has profound social implications, and is a theme that occupies me often as I add these commentaries.

It is easy to suppose that responsibility, in the Perlsian sense, means almost a freedom to belong or hang loose. I am the figure of my gestalt, and you of yours. But we are indivisible from the field. Goodman (1968) speculates about the group in a certain sense pre-dating or having more salience than the individual. Responsibility functions within the field, not extrinsically to it:

> Primitively, the ties of sex, nourishment and imitation are social but pre-personal: that is, they likely require a sense of the partners not as objects or persons, but merely as what is contacted. But at the stage of tool-making, language, and other acts of abstraction, the social functions constitute society in our special human sense: a bond among persons. The persons are formed by the social contacts they have, and they identify themselves with the social unity as a whole for their further activity.

I would like to add to this thought of Goodman's, that *a pair is itself an inter-group event*. Each partner is a group representative, whatever he or she does about it. Whatever is done will be conditioned by that group membership.

Before this afternoon no one but Pierre seems to have considered him and Orminda as a pair. Now it looks from Birde's description as if there is a general wish in the group for them to be a sexually expressed couple. It is difficult from the outside, and even more difficult for them within the group, to know yet what the group forces are in all this. The complexities they have spelled out among themselves seem grounds enough for Pierre's caution. The whole world loves a lover. There is social investment in creating pairs, for the good energy that spills round them, as well as more sombrely for the social and economic convenience of making stable pairs, more likely than isolates to conform to laws and customs, and indulge in such possibly grotesque behaviour as saddling themselves with a lifetime of mortgage debt.

Stable pairs for child-raising, in the absence of the extended family as a structure for that purpose, seem desirable at species level. But all these implications of pairing are not likely to be figural in our group.

> What is it men in women do desire?
> The lineaments of gratified desire.
> What is it women do in men desire?
> The lineaments of gratified desire.
>
> (Blake)

Perhaps this is the underlying healthy yearning in the group, expressed in this heterosexual metaphor. You search to give and exchange and be in peaceful and creative dialogue. As Birde comments, sexual behaviour may be one most potent expression of love, rather than love being a spin-off or sublimation of sexuality.

The hierarchy of gestalt formation

Perls describes a hierarchy of gestalt formation in an emergency (Perls, Hefferline and Goodman, 1961, p. 277). He was speaking of the individual. There often seems to me to be a hierarchy of gestalt formation which is related to group proximity, size, task and the law of Praegnanz. I cannot, and I daresay you yourselves cannot fully, know whether the pairs here are an expression of competition among you, or of emotional contagion, or synchronicity. Just as pairing may at times be a flight from the group, so is the small group from the large group, and so on. And isolation is a flight from all these complexities of social life.

Luckily Gestalt is less concerned with the dubious notion of causality than with existential events. What you managed here, in a way that is unusual, was to acknowledge the pairs as part of the group. I have made the point already that marriage and other long-term social pairing often serves as a substitute for, rather than a part of, belonging awarely to more complicated larger groups. Awareness of heterogeneity, and the ways we tune out or tune in various group memberships in different scenes, is to me a first task for all of us who want to make what we are learning available in more spheres than the designated therapeutic.

References

Bion W. (1961) *Experiences in Groups and Other Papers*. London: Tavistock.
Blake W. (1794) *The Complete Works of William Blake*, Ed. G. Keynes. Oxford University Press, 1966.
Cohn R. (1970) Therapy groups: psychoanalytic, experiential and Gestalt. In: J. Fagan and I.L. Shepherd (Eds), *Gestalt Therapy Now*. New York: Harper and Row, p. 134.
Daly T. (1973) From a poem written in prison.
De Mare P. (1975) In: L. Kreeger (Ed.), *The Large Group—Dynamics and Therapy*. London: Maresfield Reprints.
Goodman P. (1968) Human nature and the anthropology of neurosis. In: P.D. Pursglove (Ed.), *Recognitions in Gestalt Therapy*. New York: Funk and Wagnall, p. 75.
Jung C. (1959) Archetypes and the Collective Unconscious. In: *Collected Works*, Vol. 9. New York: Pantheon.
Merleau-Ponty M. (1962) *The Phenomenology of Perception*, Trans. C. Smith. London: Routledge.
Miller E. and Rice A. (1967) *Systems of Organization*. London: Tavistock.
Perls F., Hefferline R. and Goodman P. (1961) *Gestalt Therapy*. New York: Dell.

Plato. *Symposium*, Trans. Hamilton Walter (1951). Harmondsworth: Penguin.
Schutz W. (1960) *Firo: A Three-Dimensional Theory of Interpersonal Behaviour*. New York: Holt, Rinehart and Winston.
Simmel G. (1950) *The Sociology of Georg Simmel*, Ed. K. Wolff. New York: The Free Press.

Chapter 10

Wednesday evening: Destructuring or destruction

Jan writes: Maybe you are as cohesive a group tonight as you people will ever get to be. And too you seem right out on that edge between the Second Law of Thermodynamics, entropy, and Anti-Chaos Theory, the tendency to organisation and growth. The title I put to your session seems a strong theme, though its polarities are there too. De-structuring, taking experience to bits as we take food to bits when chewing (Perls 1947), is a favourite notion in Gestalt. It suggests that potential nourishment can then be retained, and translated into new forms before being assimilated.

The processes of change can be subtle or violent, quick or slow, bonfire or compost. The essential is whether I can then re-combine, re-integrate into functional new forms. And I guess that fear of destruction can inhibit de-structuring. Grace gives us evidence of this when she holds back, and suspects others of holding back, in saying all they want to Manfred about his going.

You are faced tonight with, among much else, the beginning of group disintegration as Manfred prepares to leave. At times it sounds as if there is a belief that the group is some kind of milk-jug, which will be irreversibly broken by his going. There is also some fear that he will be broken, or at least suffer considerably. It looks likely that the fear he generated earlier in the week is still present enough to keep anyone except Sappho from confronting him about this. Whether this omission is destructive may be considered. Whether his indulging his feelings for Annie would in another way be destructive or constructive is considered, by Grace at least.

It appears that she did not circulate this report until the week was over. This once more raises the question of whether withholding is destructive, since it gives no material for de-structuring.

Grace's account

Loss was around for me before we even sat down together in the library. You've told me I'm too cocky, Jan, in my smooth dissimulating way. That tendency has taken a knock. And I remember that old German professor at Stanford, shouting at me, "It is very important to fail! It is so dangerous to be always successful! How grows the immune system without exposure to disease!" I didn't fail much in those days. The black girl from Britain on a Fulbright. And sexy with it. I have to tell this before I can go on with the He Said She Said business about this evening.

Since I was about eleven I have just loved sex, and just loved sexual appreciation: thirty-five years on one drug. It's hard to bust the habit. Those words sound so flip. More of my smooth dissimulating.

I've done three catty things in this group: getting Orminda to confess her negative feelings for her mother-in-law, to the group; messing up the time boundary with Manfred one day; sniping at Pierre. I suppose I shall just have to take my punishment.

Pierre could be an amazing lover, even if, as I suspect, he is not at the moment. And I want to Svengali him. I want him. I want that complicated mind and that brilliance. I could handle his petulance. I hurt, Jan. I hated this first experience of being passed over. And in the group I said nothing of that. I thought it was to do with protecting Orminda. I think too it was that I was too proud, and that I had no immune defences prepared.

I don't look forty-six. Having those fibroids is the only sign I've had of age. I look twenty-eight. I want to be twenty-eight all the time, so I'm the *jeunesse qui peut* as well as *la vieillesse qui sait*. I feel undermined, uncertain, destroyed, at being relegated to the wallflower line of middle-aged women who are not lusted after in this group. And even Annie had Manfred confessing the hots for her.

Destructuring or destruction 133

O God. The new age woman who turns out to define herself by her relationship to men in true traditional fashion. Now it feels a bit as if I have allowed myself a long, insensate scream. Now I feel more connected.

We were more sombre at supper than usual, though whether because of all the pairing stuff or just from absolute exhaustion from last night, I can't tell. Sappho suggested that we were tired, and should take the evening off and go our own ways. Annie pointed out that it would be our last evening with Manfred. Well wouldn't she?

"If he is not busy with his other friends," said Sappho. When he said that he was expecting to be with us, she answered that that was what she had expected last night, but had not got. Birde urged that we all meet, saying something that did not exactly turn me on, about a ceremony of farewell. There was obviously a task of reparation for the group. But I had my own wounds to lick. And Sappho had pursed lips, Sohan and Chuck were vague and star-struck, and Pierre in what is becoming his normal state of deathly pallor.

I'm grateful now that Birde and Annie made us meet. We actually assembled at nine o'clock, half an hour later than we had agreed. And even then, Manfred was a few seconds later than everyone else. Bizarre.

We started with what felt like the version of Musical Chairs they might play in Hell, it was so painful to me. Pierre sat down between Sohan and Chuck. Sappho made Birde move up so she could sit next to Chuck. Then he got up and came and sat near Orminda. I wanted so much to join in and push between her and Pierre so that I was near him. But I sat there in bad faith (Sartre 1943); false to my real needs. When Manfred entered, attention to the seating plan made everyone watch for his move, almost without breathing. Annie was sitting between Chuck and Birde. Would he sit beside her? Would he choose the side which placed him between her and Birde, or the other side, near his friend Chuck? Or would he go for the electrically-charged place for any man in the group tonight, beside Orminda?

Whether systems training, tact or sheer unwatchful serendipity won, he sat in the place I thought best, between Annie and Birde. I had Sohan between me and Pierre, which meant that I did not need to meet Pierre's eyes, for which I was thankful.

We sat in silence and I felt angry with everyone for wasting time. The tape is self-explanatory, once the voices start.

SOHAN: If I may ask, I should like to know at what time tomorrow Manfred will be leaving us?
BIRDE: It's such a shame! Can't you ring your wife now, Manfred, and arrange to meet her on Friday afternoon? You're part of the group now. We can't let you go.
MANFRED: I leave in the morning.
BIRDE: But when you arrived you hadn't planned to walk out before the end. Surely she can look after herself for one day. There's time to ring her now. Hasn't she got friends or anything she can see?
ORMINDA: Bargaining with death.
PIERRE: It is my impression that the beginning of the session is the moment of disclosures.
CHUCK: The floor is yours.
PIERRE: Perhaps all there is to disclose is great fatigue and a wish to go early to bed.
SOHAN: Oo. [*He kind of groaned*].
MANFRED: Have you sickness?
SAPPHO: Nobody has admired my skirt. It is from India, like you, Sohan.
SOHAN: O yes, very admirable.

At this point Annie suddenly erupted and told Sappho to take her skirt and stuff it in her mouth by way of gag, rather than use it to gag other people as she just had. It's true that Sappho is for ever cutting in with some observation about her fascinating self, so I kind of lose whatever else is going on. Annie, I suspect buoyed up by Manfred's sexual appreciation, took charge and asked Sohan what he had groaned about. He admitted that when bed was mentioned, he had thought of what after some discussion we established as the Great Bed of Ware, which he thought he had seen in the Victoria and Albert Museum. There was some rueful kind of laughter. But the taboo was broken, at least, about mentioning the pairs which had suddenly, from being the open topic in the last session, gone underground.

Brooding silence once more. Then Manfred said, "Annie, all shall be well". His voice sounded almost priestly, gentle, as he

Destructuring or destruction

looked across at Annie and said some words that seemed like a blessing, a reassurance at a funeral, at once poignant and comforting. He sat very still, poised, more a man than I had ever seen him. He gave presence to what he was saying. Or perhaps what he was saying gave him presence.

Annie looked at him and flushed slowly, so I could see the blood go up her neck into her face, till even her forehead was pink. She said something about making an end being also a beginning.

At first I thought he was speaking some lines from the Bible. Now I began to recall fragments of The Four Quartets (Eliot 1944). The words seemed swollen with meaning. They seemed to stand for so much that was not being said between the two of them. Pierre looked at the floor and kept stroking his right hand with his left. Yeah. He was more or less out of my sight lines, but I know every movement he made. There was quiet for a time. Then out of the blue Birde said that she had heard that another larger group was arriving at the barn block in the morning. There was disjointed talk about it being a funny time of week to start a group. I asked what was going on. Chuck made what must be one of his first extended process comments.

"Birde was talking about change, I guess. Manfred is going, so we're making some kind of an ending. And into that comes a new group that will probably pull this one together no end."

Annie said by way of comment, with a nanosecond of a smile, another line of poetry. I don't know what she was quoting from, but she and Manfred looked at each other again. It is extraordinary that he knows so much English literature. Sohan shifted about and cleared his throat and said:

"I am thinking, how are we still this group when Manfred goes? Yes, yes, I am sure we are. But it is strange. And if one other comes, perhaps Jan, I think we are still this group. Perhaps to others this is not strange. But in this moment I marvel that what is not the same also is the same."

"If seven of us left and a different seven came, would it be the same group then?" asked Birde. The talk circled around the pace of change people guessed was assimilable. Pierre said we were defending ourselves from the change that was happening here. Orminda said we were chewing and trying to digest the change that was happening here. He agreed with her. It was quite unnerving to see this hyena lie down with the lamb. And he did not appear to capitulate or throw away his argument, but just to listen to hers with the sort of attention I hope he gives his clients, but which he rarely shows us, his peers.

More quiet, as the poem words about ends and beginnings flowed into Sohan's. As I asked myself whether Annie and Manfred would spend the night together; whether Pierre and Orminda would spend the night together; whether Sappho would shanghai Chuck into bed with her. I confess it, I even found myself in a momentary tenderness and lust towards Sohan. Your training has shown me the likely transferential nature of that. Sohan as an understudy for Pierre suggests a certain desperation in the beholder's eye.

Birde spoke beautifully into the quiet. She said she wanted to help make a farewell, or witness a farewell to Manfred, but kept finding herself with images of his leave-taking being from Annie more than the rest of us. He nodded, looking ready to cry. I felt anxious at the thought of this rigid man, who has been through such a spiritual upheaval in the last day and night, going back into tourist London with a perhaps nagging wife. Many of us nodded. Manfred said,

> ... "we by a love so much refined
> That ourselves know not what it is"...

Annie continued, seemingly unwilling,

> ... "Inter-assured of the mind
> Care less eyes, lips and hands to miss."

Manfred quoted more Donne, from *The Second Anniversary*

> "Her pure and innocent blood
> Spoke in her cheeks, and so distinctly wrought
> That one might also say, her body thought."

I've been struggling lately with how to modify that Cycle of Experience model, to take account of reciprocity and field more demonstrably. Suddenly something Sonia Nevis said to a group of us last year about waves and particles, formed into a clear image. I saw Annie and Manfred in wave form, instead of being separate particles. They were making a simultaneous wave, their boundaries forming one. The wave was strengthening from their simultaneity, and making a great arc, almost visible to me in the room, as the rest of us made, I think, the same shape of wave, Greek chorusing below the height of their peaks. It was not the moment to talk of this insight. Maybe, in the intensity of the field we were forming, other people were sparked into great inner satoris. The strangeness of it all was that this meeting between Annie and Manfred was so cryptic, expressed in borrowed lines, with the most fleeting eye contact. Manfred's cheek and one side of his mouth trembled. Annie had tears in her eyes. There was every sign of the strength of boundary disturbance happening to each. Their contact was up at I–Thou intensity.

One way, I can say, all right, that was the creation of the we. The group empathy seemed palpable.

Manfred slapped his thighs very softly, seeming intent on remembering some more lines. He held his arms oddly, so what he did was pointed at his sex. I noticed, then looked at other people, and saw them looking straight at his hands too. He said a verse I recognised from the Song of Solomon:

"Until the day break, and the shadows flee away, turn, by beloved, and be like a roe or a young hart upon the mountains of Bethel."

He allowed himself his ration of one look at Annie, and she looked back at him, saying steadily:

"By night on my bed I sought him, him whom my soul loveth."

She paused, and added:

"I sought him, but I found him not."

Sappho broke across the quiet to say crossly that she did not know the words and did not understand, and felt excluded. Her sphere had not exactly moved into wave form. Here were two passionate inhibited people, expressing love in a way I imagine was totally novel and yet totally comprehensible to both. But young Narcissus was jealous.

Orminda said that she could not understand the words completely, but felt moved nevertheless. Pierre agreed quickly. When did Pierre ever agree quickly with anyone before? He spoke of the sound of the words, and the magical linkage of the two voices as they remembered the quotations. He said that intellectual comprehension could be a barrier to experience. Pierre! But that is what I want in him, Jan. That is what I am mourning now. He has depth, he has insight, he has these sudden descents into humility from his know-allness. Manfred looked up at him, I think gratefully, and said more lines of poetry. I have looked since, and know they were the last lines of T. S. Eliot's "Burnt Norton". I felt the pang of some words about the waste sad time before and after. And there was that paradox of here, now and always that is the poetry behind what we debase into the humdrum of Gestalt technique.

But now I felt excluded. They were in deeper water than I could swim in. Or was it that Pierre was pairing with Manfred, not me? Both.

This time when there was silence it felt awkward: I was sitting there retroflecting, censoring questions and comments, even complaints that were coming up in me about moving up into the stratosphere, some mystery region where we were all losing sight of the ground. Orminda spoke for me, but with thoughts put together in a way mine were not.

"What in the name of heaven are you all on about? Well I'll tell you, without any of your half-guessed bloody hints. There's Manfred who's done some magician's trick on us, of growing up from being the bad boy of the lower fourth, into the hero of the school, eighteen years old and at the height of his sexual powers according to the Gospel of Masters and Johnson. And Annie's this fifteen year old who doesn't know her arse from her elbow when it comes to conducting a carnal affair. Incarnation, that was the word in that poem of yours. Carnality's nearer the mark." She paused briefly, than added, "And there's no need for the any of youse to be pointing out the projective element in my remarks." There was an almost hysterical amount of laughing. Annie agreed that she felt fifteen. Chuck agreed that he felt adolescent. We sort of got it together that as a group we felt adolescent, and with it all, parental to each other, so we were bothered about Manfred's going off into the world too early.

Looking back, I know this was a euphemism for voicing this

Destructuring or destruction

doubt about the world he was going back to. But I did not say it. Nobody did. Pierre made the observation, to the air, that chastity was a very proper solution to the sexual temptations of adolescence. For a moment I felt a stab of glee, because that sounded as if he meant that no one would have him. Half a second later I felt angry with his primness, and wanted Orminda comforted by his body in her bed. I wanted him shaken up, too.

Chuck said that Manfred going felt to him like a rehearsal of the death of the group. He said he wanted his death to be like this—living hard till the last moment. Manfred really listened to him. Jan, it's ridiculous how I construed everything in terms of the act of sex. I heard Chuck's words as advice that he and Annie should be carnal, and Manfred's listening as acceptance. This too goes by the name of projection.

I need a partner who's my own size, and who'll commit himself to me, and who I'll commit to. Which takes me back to Pierre.

I stopped writing for a while. Coming back to the group, I remember, without turning the tape on, that Annie suddenly looked white. The word death had perhaps done it. She said, after twice opening her mouth silently, as if her spirit was not up to the pain of what she was going to say:

> *"All familiar things he touched,*
> *All common words he spake, became to me*
> *Like forms and sounds of a diviner world.*
> *As terrible and lovely as a tempest:*
> *He came, and went, and left me what I am."*

I thought straightaway of me and Pierre, not wanting this epitaph of Shelley's to be ours. Surprisingly, Sohan picked up the dialogue here:

"I think it is the only time in my life I have been present in the forming of these strong attachments between people, while being allowed to take part in the pair in more ways than to say only congratulations and so on. Now I have a most strong sense of appreciation of Manfred, and great admiring that he has warm feelings for Annie, who is all parts of him he needs, I think." The wisdom of what he was saying poked awkwardly through his words, like a gift wrapped in a lump of old newspaper. "And I hope earnestly that in looking at the pair we do not forget to make our farewells with Manfred all as a group. In my art classes sometimes we place a paper on the back of a leaving member, on which all may write messages, with or without signatures."

I felt embarrassed at this suggestion. Now I think it was a good one. Nobody else demurred, anyway. The effect was that Manfred was made central, physically, and let himself submit to our scrawlings. In writing we touched him, and that felt good. And he was left with a testament, which I reckon for someone as inept at hearing good messages as he is, to be a good thing. Sappho took the paper off his back when all had written, rolled it up and gave it to him, with some theatrical panache. That, oddly, felt right too. If Annie had done it, the sub-system would have been separate again. Sappho needs—the phrase comes to me from the title of a film—she needs to be a member of the wedding.

I stuck my oar in, and asked Manfred if he had any other ideas of what he needed before we stopped. He closed his eyes, then opened them and got up, and went round the circle, shaking hands with people and saying thank you. When he came to Annie she stood up. He shook hands with her too, then gave her a snatched kiss on the cheek. Sappho commented the gracelessness of his movement. Annie very slowly opened her arms a little away from her body. He felt his chin as if to test the stubble growth, then said thank you again, and that he must pack. Aborted energy. There's a line somewhere in Adrian Mitchell about wanting a world where people can go about freely, and make love freely.

Yes Jan, I know, it would not work. Female sexual energy is out of kilter with the male. It's no good pretending that in an ideal world Orminda could have Pierre and I could too. He'd be dead in a week.

And the joke does not stop me tormenting myself, remembering where I last saw Pierre and Orminda, at the door of his room, in deep talk.

I keep thinking of Sonia Nevis tonight, and her question, "Does it matter?" She says that word with such passion and energy. Yes it matters, Sonia. And what matters is love being expressed. My hurt pride is to do with my competitiveness, and with a shortage of resources. I do have some love for Orminda and for Pierre, so I want their freedom, finally, more than I want to possess him. But it's kind of a close thing.

Destructuring or destruction

So this is the egocentric way I finish the story of an evening that was centrally to do with our leaving ceremony. But I am showing, I think, the mood of the group at the end of the evening. There was a melting away, accompanied with beady furtive looks from me at who was going where with whom. Tomorrow we'll see whether the pairs have destroyed the group, and whether the indifference to each other I sensed at moments in myself tonight is the beginning of the loosening and disintegration and withdrawal into the death of the group. You would call it post-contact, when we have partly digested each other into our physiology, partly reinforced the way we are already, by rejecting the models round us. There is a great uneasiness in me, that I need to find new ways of being in the world. If I matter enough.

Then the weird idea comes to me that the pairs might be a desperate bid for life and the immortality of this shared bit of life.

Jan's comment

It would be easy to sit and speculate on what Manfred may be up to in going, and what the rest of you are up to in keeping your persuading of him to stay till the eleventh hour, when his wife is presumably on her way, and he is perhaps less likely to change plans again. I wonder instead on whether you have all been players in a repeated destructive pattern in his life and yours, or whether this was a startling episode for most of you, which will be digested into new behaviour, rather than serve to reinforce old prejudices. Such one-sided dialogue could soon land me in a theory quagmire.

I turn to what seems to me firmer ground, an idea which occurs to me time and again in small group work. Mourning is one of the many forms of emotional de-structuring and assimilation which often seem to me more economically achieved by the group than by the individual alone. The tasks or likely responses in mourning, are shared around the group. Sappho does the bargaining, when she tries at the beginning to persuade Manfred to stay longer. By the end of the evening, it is not clear from Grace's account whether she is alone in carrying depression for the group. Perhaps she is, and perhaps some of those who may have gone off into pairs are going through denial, another aspect of mourning. Annie seems to be the most open channel of pure grief at the loss of him. It is easy to think of her as a widow at this moment, for all the transience and unexpressedness of the meeting between her and Manfred. The lines of poetry became the expression of transcendence, of the illumination or satori that can be there in passionate experience fully lived. The rest of the group look trustworthy as comforters, when she needs them.

Perhaps what have to be stages of mourning within one person have happened alongside each other, in the co-operative work of the group. They do the work in front of each other, so take from and add to the composite.

Reading Grace's account has taken me back to T. S. Eliot, and I think of those lines near the end of "East Coker", which say that the world grows stranger, the pattern, the gestalt, more complicated, as we grow older. Moments are not isolated: now and now and now. The whole of my life and many lives before mine, is present in each moment. Everything I want to teach about the importance of every action, about responsibility, about awareness, is summed up for me.

There is a sense of continuity and universality in these lines. There is also a feeling of vastness, that might overwhelm or at least daunt an individual. As part of a group, I suggest that the members can allow themselves into greater intensity and greater perspective in their experience, in an economy of time. The processes of mourning illustrate this, often with particular clarity.

The group this evening suggests the image of a container, robust enough to contain the very processes of destructuring. Earlier on, I remember Manfred being gloomy about the imposition of meaning on what may be meaningless. Now it is he who gives poetic value and meaning to what seems the anguish of his under-expressed relation to Annie and the group. The jug is not broken. Yet. With sexual arousal the valency of the group, a fragmentation may be to come. Now thoughts of Freud (1920) and a masochistic death instinct, of Kohut (1977, p. 133) and triumphant death, jostle my own pedestrian annoyance that Perls, Hefferline and Goodman did not sound a clear trumpet note about all the phases of individual and group life.

Gestalt Therapy (1951) shows awareness of the phases of life, but a refusal to categorise and relate them in any detail. The field of psychological theory in which Perls and Goodman emerged gave such enormous attention to categorisation of personality, aberrant behaviour, ages and stages and so forth, that these two writers' insistence on the particular made an important point. The vigour and creativity of childhood is prized by the writers. The post-contact phase of relinquishing and dying in old age is less mentioned. Here the work of Freud (1921), Stern (1985), Winnicott (1964), Skynner and Cleese (1983), Bales (1970) and a great number of other theorists who have focussed attention on the possible recapitulation of personal development in group development, form a compatible extension to Gestalt theory. What Gestalt points up with marvellous clarity is the creative possibility inherent but not inevitable in destructuring. It's up to me what I make of it. I can make it and you and me matter.

References

Bales R. (1970) *Personality and Interpersonal Behaviour*. New York: Rinehart and Winston.
Eliot T.S. (1944) *The Four Quartets*. London: Faber and Faber.
Freud S. (1920) *Beyond the Pleasure Principle*. Standard Ed. London: Hogarth Press, 1955.
Freud S. (1921) *Group Psychology and the Analysis of the Ego*. Standard Ed. London: Hogarth Press, 1955.
Kohut H. (1977) *The Restoration of the Self*. Madison: International Universities Press.
Perls F.S. (1947) *Ego, Hunger and Aggression*. New York: Random House.
Perls F.S., Hefferline R. and Goodman P. (1951) *Gestalt Therapy*. Excitement and Growth in the Human Personality. New York: Julian Press.
Sartre J-P. (1943) *L'Etre et Le Neant*. Paris: Gallimard.
 Sartre proposed the simple idea that at any time each of us is either acting in good faith, which is in line with an inner sense of what is right for us at the moment, or in bad faith, which is the opposite. Perls and Goodman were influenced by various aspects of Existentialism.
Skynner R. and Cleese J. (1983) *Families and How to Survive Them*. London: Methuen.
Stern D. (1985) *The Interpersonal World of the Infant*. New York: Basic Books.
Winnicott (1964) *The Child, the Family and the Outside World*. Harmondsworth: Penguin.

Chapter 11

Thursday morning: New configurations

Jan writes: With the group death stalking near, there are perceptible changes of mode and content in the group, it seems to me. Manfred has gone; I am no better than an illusion. The world outside the group looms into awareness, maybe against your will. The response is both to meet it, and to close ranks into an affective haven within the group. I think of Gustafson and Cooper (1990), saying

> ...in securing organisation, one must evoke a sense of Us and Them. The Dynamic forces of cohesiveness and alliance draw the common antagonist into clarity. Within the sharpness of Us and Them great power and accomplishment can be generated. Since these are changeable social forces, one must be prepared to monitor misuse and falseness.

The new configurations show in Annie herself, as well as in the larger field.

Annie's account

The unspoken decision was that we had the first phase of the group over the breakfast table. There were probably four or five of us present when Chuck came into the room singing, *"There were eight in the bed, and the little one said, Roll over, roll over."*

New configurations

I was glad that he could be so ridiculous about Manfred's going. There is a flesh wound in me from that, but not more. And I want to be over it. I am still hurt, narcissistically, that Manfred did not change his nature and sleep with me last night. Looking at him with judgement, I imagine how disastrous it would have been to him to do so. And for goodness sake, would I have wanted Manfred round my neck for life, with his sniffy obsessional high handed ways?

There, I am doing my best to wash him out of my hair. And that's mostly to do with getting up at six this morning and knowing from the cold kettle that he had not been down already. I stood with a cup of coffee at the front door. I told myself I was being in the here and now, enjoying the dawn freshness of a day that looked set to be cloudlessly hot within a couple of hours. I smelled the thick scent of the jasmine, and looked at the early bees in the hollyhocks that grow up through the cracks of the terrace.

By eight o'clock I was ready to cry. I went up to his room, and opened the door when he did not answer my knock. Cold bed. No luggage. God knows when he must have tiptoed off. I hated him.

Birde came down late, which is not typical of her, and Sappho did not arrive till after nine. So there was plenty of room for us at the table, where we sat talking over the cooling teapot and bent toast. Manfred's disappearance without farewells was mentioned with care. I was the one who said that it was easier to understand him clinically than to feel very drawn to him as a companion. I am glad that no one joined in what I might have turned to a spiteful re-working of history. Grace and Sohan and Orminda had come down early, on purpose to see him off, so they must have been sore too.

Casually, Grace said Jan had been on the phone to say he was in bed with food-poisoning. We murmured perfunctory regret.

Sohan reminded us that there was to be another whole community meeting in the afternoon, at which we should be the smallest group. An ecology conference is arriving this morning, to the far barn block, which I had just thought was an empty farm building. There will be about thirty of them. There was quite a strong move in our group to miss the meeting.

Tomorrow we shall leave. So we are a bit irrelevant to the place now. I notice the superficial way I am recording this. The underlying motive is to normalise, to explain away, to blur.

Orminda was flowering this morning, nourished by the adoration of many men, I think. Her eyes looked bigger, her features nearer the edges of her face, somehow. When she came she was pinched in. She is perhaps our group success. She was restless with ideas energy, and had the look of understanding to the roots whatever was before her. She looked at her plate for a minute while the rest of us were persuading ourselves out of the community meeting, and then began to talk. There was no tape recorder on, so I have to recall as I can what she said. I remember specially how she kept half-standing, then sitting again, as if her insights needed her to get up and act on them straightaway.

"Over and over, the choice is between staying home and rubbing along or scuffling along, or working as a group to meet the next group. Time was, the Unions had some support from membership. Then that went to such a degree that the Union leaders were a separate entity, negotiating with the bosses, without the backing of the membership. So the opening was there for Government to come in and take away their powers. Power is potentially in the most numerous group (Brown 1978). Divide and rule. And it all starts with sitting around the table, sitting around the canteen for another fag and a gossip, instead of finding out how to be a united front, and an intelligent front."

Grace sang, "*As soon as this pub closes, The revolution starts.*" The second musical contribution. Birde, who had just come down, asked hesitantly what there was for us to present a united front about here.

"About the making of a good history," said Orminda, with weight. "Think of it. There is an unbroken continuity built into these community meetings here."

"I see these meetings in one chain over many years, perhaps into the next century," said Sohan. People demurred about breaks at Christmas and holiday times, and Pierre interrupted:

"These rationalisations are perhaps once more the way we sit and gossip, making comfortable pastimes within the group, rather than internalise, as Sohan has done, the idea Orminda offers us."

"And you, in one sentence, both express your feelings for Orminda, and support this move towards aware contact between groups, as well as between individuals," said Grace. She sounded as if she was learning as she spoke.

"The ability to over-determine is what can make angels or idiots of the human race," said Pierre to her. I felt that he was pairing with her in a way that was good for both of them. Words are the symbols by which they will make their best contacts.

Responses to the large group

Stumblingly, we all began to confess the forms of our resistance to meeting the other groups. The feeling was of each person reaching large insights, and applying them, not just inwards, but as outsight too.

I know I label the other groups stupid. Sohan said he told himself that his English would not be clear enough for them; and he saw how this was a retroflection of a judgement that they would not be good enough for him. Sappho said she regressed, in the intergroup scene, to one of her ways of going on as a fourth child. She fights for attention, in panic that the larger the number present, the less attention she may be allowed. She linked this to her choice of profession, the perpetual stardom of being a psychodrama director.

Pierre spoke with energetic self-castigation of the contempt he could direct at any out-group, recalling his derision of the smelliness and hairiness of some of the counsellors. Sappho pointed out how seven-year-old this reaction was, from such an insightful process commentator. As usual, he reacted with what looked like enjoyment of his ability to be destructive and infantile. It is an endearing *faiblesse*.

"Et voila," said Pierre, with his little shrug, "To see much is to see much. It is not the same as to be mature." Suddenly he looked most dejected. I thought to myself that from the look of him, he had certainly not got over his scruples and slept with Orminda last night. There was a little silence round the table, and I suppose other people may have been coming to the same kinds of opinion, and containing them as I did.

Birde contributed that she anaesthetises herself in large groups. She cannot think of them as inter-group events. She loses all group identity and feels isolated and powerless (Turquet 1975). Chuck, looking animated, slapped his leg and guffawed, mocking himself, as he explained how he had just realised that he stores much of his aggressive energy when he is at work, and brings it out in big meetings where he is The Medical Representative. He wants to beat the hell out of the other groups (Gustafson and Cooper 1989). Then he is left being the prime mover, apparently responsible for the whole outcome of the meeting, which was not what he wanted at all. The contrast with Birde was striking, and made all of us notice our tendency to be all or nothing in the face of big meetings.

Most of us agreed that we put ourselves at the nothing end of the spectrum, particularly by avoiding the meetings altogether whenever possible.

Orminda brought us back to now, and said more about her vision of an evolution, a gradual acculturation in this conference centre, which we would inevitably influence. She reminded us of the Polsters' definition of three forms of contact: *intrapersonal, interpersonal* and what they call *international*, by which they mean that each group actually listens to the other (Polster 1987). Birde, not listening, said:

"As you speak I think again of all who have lived and died in this house, over centuries. Then this lady we do not know was moved to dedicate it to groups like ours. Her now was formed by all that past, I think, as she did it. And from our little time here, we have reached this moment, when we make a new sense of our bad behaviours at the last community meeting." I remembered and quoted the opening of "Burnt Norton" (Eliot 1936). Just as last night, a poet could do a better job for me than I could myself, or than Birde could in her fumblings in a foreign language. I wondered if she and the others had been angry at that strange exchange last night between Manfred and me, of lines I had not even known I could remember. But she smiled across at me brilliantly, recognising in Eliot's words some of what she had been trying to say.

We were back in our dialogue in which we meet each other's desire, and find words to express something that is being created by all of us. I think of the dramatic conventions which say that there is little excitement without conflict. There is huge conflict, or at least huge struggle, in working to enter each other's worlds and admit them for our own. The fight is against incomprehension, which bedevils all our communicating.

New configurations

"So much power," said Grace, sounding tired. "We can skip the meeting and have a swim, and so deny continuity. Or we can turn up and find a way to deal with the new group coming in as cackhanded and bolshie as we were the other day."

"I so wish to swim again," said Birde wistfully.

"O no! I will not tolerate these martyrdoms," said Sappho. "We have time to swim and also time to go to the meeting."

Sohan said urgently, "It is after ten o'clock, and I have uneasy feelings. I am most engaged in our talk here. But never before have we had our meeting round the food table. The breakfast is still here. We have not made our disclosures. I do not think we have appointed anyone to record. Somehow I connect all this to the going of Manfred."

I agreed with him. "We're being sloppy in a way he would not have allowed?"

Pierre went on, "And also the group teaches me to be as you say sloppy. We abandon the structure we agreed, and I have the thought, What does it matter? What does it matter if I betray my beliefs about proper conduct in the group, my beliefs about proper conduct in marriage?" He sounded as if it all mattered a great deal. I offered:

"Perhaps sitting like this is very useful to us just now. We are close together and facing in. And we have had what I think is one of the most illuminating conversations I can remember, about shifts of consciousness inside each one of us, when we are aware of the environment at inter-group level. We have talked about processes that can stay locked inside people, unexamined. So now we can make a shift if we wish to, with awareness."

The small group again

"And sitting with a table between us makes us into these safe animals who relate to each other above the waist," said Orminda, again not sounding enamoured of the safety she was describing. "Centaurs with the horse bit hidden (Erikson 1964). I scared myself stiff yesterday with that extraordinary openness about pairing. Part of the scare was of being torn to pieces by the women, because of the way the transferences worked out."

Several voices protested and heckled her for this form of words. She went on, "And then there was the fear that the group would splinter to bits. Maybe God got that worry, when he allowed separate consciousness in each person. We'd lose the sense of the whole, of being part of the whole. Sorry God. We did." She paused, reflecting, and we waited for her. She went on, "And there was another fear, that I have again now. It's of too much. It's of letting in so much insight that..."

She stopped again, and Pierre prompted her quietly, "That what? That you will be flooded with total insight, and with an anguish of feeling that is insupportable for one human being?" She nodded.

Grace said doggedly, "You are talking about yourself, Pierre." He nodded. I felt very tenderly towards her, for working to further the dialogue of love that struggled for a channel between Pierre and Orminda. This was group consciousness, to me. With unpossessive love she was leaving this sub-system intact, but not falling into the tacitness that so easily occurs around pairs within a group.

Birde said, "It is time for us to clear the breakfast, then go and meet without a table to guard our private parts." There was a release of screeching, tense laughter at her words. We all got up straightaway and set about what she had suggested.

Although it was so glorious outside, we met in a rather dark room I called the linenfold room, because of the carving on the panelling which lined it. It felt a little like a conspirator's room. That is the first comment I have on the tape. Chuck said it, and Pierre countersuggested, "To me it resembles the priests's confessional box."

"So the plot is about how to be better people," said Grace. Time and again, her voice chimes in right after Pierre's. Maybe that is the last trace of her contest with Orminda for possession of him. But I will not erase what I have already written to the opposite effect. I think both are true.

Now I will edit away many of these mini satori that happen every few seconds now. The main work of the morning was truly, I think, to plan before going to the community meeting in the afternoon. Birde suggested that we start by confessing the bad feelings we had had or still had. Chuck said we should not sit in one block, as that presented a threatening front to the rest. We all puzzled about the ways in which we could manipulate or manage the conduct of the group meeting. It sounds obvious now. But I had sudden clarity as we were talking, about needing to know what

New configurations 151

meetings are for, before arriving at them. I struggled to convey this, and people heard me.

"This is the excellence of psychodrama," said Sappho, inevitably. "All understand they are there for the self-exploration in a supportive environment."

"And that is the limitation of these programmatic methods," Pierre replied. "It is most agreeable to wallow on the sunbed of the contrived supportive group. And how thus does any member explore the here and now of envy, spite, hate, all that is not allowed in this massage parlour of the psyche?" Grace gave him a verbal cuff for this slanted view of Sappho's work. This did not stop Sappho from being very angry. Chuck said:

"He says he's destructive, Sappho. You don't have to join in the game and let him be. As long as you strive to win that little skirmish with him, you're not putting your energy into the whole war strategy." Birde objected to the idea of war.

Sohan said, "The war is against unawareness, against the poverty of ways we have to be full people in these larger settings such as will be this afternoon." I was privately amazed at the sophistication of his thinking. Orminda took his hand and smiled into his eyes. Maybe he was one of Plato's army, producing more than his best, in order to be the better adored by his beloved.

Now now. I said that I would simply report our main strategic plan. Yet all this was of it. Chuck's comment on Sappho's part in allowing Pierre to be a pest was taken up and talked of at length, by both of them as well as the rest of us.

"This is the psychodynamics," said Pierre. "The force goes out from subject to object. And here the Gestalt observation is the more useful. The nature of the contact is the vital here. From this comes stagnation, repetition or the creative breakthrough. And for this, both parties are needed."

"Too fast, too fast," said Orminda. "There's no time to digest. Now let's go back. We need to know what the meeting is for, if we're to have any idea what to do at it. What's the outcome we want?"

I suggested it was hierarchical, in the sense that the older group were momentarily the priests of the place, handing on a history and an ethos to the novitiates entering. Orminda kept Sappho from butting in with another idea, until this one had been assimilated.

In Gestalt language, we chewed it over thoroughly. It looked to me as if we all became priests as we talked. We sat more upright and spoke in a more measured way. We gave up the excited interruptive style that had erupted from time to time earlier on. The weight of history was on us, and the responsibility of colouring the future.

"I remember," said Birde, "a training I was in in Sweden. The senior year to us were the first ever to take that training. At the time of their graduation, they informed us that it was a tradition that the lower year should make a party for the people leaving. We were so angry, and felt so powerless! Of course it was a lie that there could be a tradition. We felt their attempt at overpowering us, and soon we were the successful underdogs, forgetting to buy the alcohol, burning the food, and feeling tired and leaving the party."

"That's what got hierophants a bad name," said Chuck. "Abuse of the system. Unilateral tradition is out, then."

"But this is most illuminating," said Pierre. "This is the problem. Tradition appears to be unilateral, to belong to the old ones and be imposed on the young. And the function of the rebelliousness of youth is to test the tradition, to see if it merits to be conserved."

"And to see if it can be chewed through and re-personalised, owned by the new generation."

"At a Gestalt conference a speaker made a description in Gestalt terms of four ways we treat the new, the novel (Knopf, 1991). One way was only to use the new figure to excite the boundaries, without letting it in to be assimilated. This is the danger this afternoon, that we offer such wonderful insights and ethoses, and the new group do as we did at the beginning of the week. Certainly we got excited, but only to mock and reject. So adolescent," said Birde.

"And the way we did that will colour how the counsellor group feel towards us this afternoon," said Orminda. We were all quiet, maybe wondering again whether it would not be a better use of our time to take a hedonistic solution by swimming in the stream, and forgetting the meeting entirely.

"There is a major choice," said Pierre, "Of whether to see the meeting as an experience of process, and to comment on the phenomenology of that as we observe it; or to attempt to manage the meeting, so that we attempt at least to impose what will happen."

"And there's the intermediate position," said Orminda, "in which

New configurations

we maybe tell our dilemma and the awareness that's come out of it, and suggest a structure." I and Sohan did not follow what she meant, so she explained. "For example we could say that we need help in working out a way of making these meetings as productive and flexible as possible. For me, that's simply the truth."

"And also this melts the resistance. It invites the collaboration," said Pierre. She nodded and went on, "Then we could suggest that we break into sub-groups of three or four, formed of all three groups present. Each of them could find what they needed to do and say for about ten or fifteen minutes, then make a paper to show their findings. Then the sub-groups could pair, to double in size and compare and expand their findings. Their task could be to report back by producing another paper to the whole group. It's not original, for goodness' sake. It's just effective. Everyone gets a say. And the content is not too heavily conditioned by the process." We got into a lively discussion of how long should be allowed to each phase, and whether a silent time should precede.

Grace interrupted to say, "I like the idea, and I've got faith in it. But no way is having a smart idea going to prevent inter-group rivalrous feelings. Look what we're doing. We're cornering power, even if it is supposed to be for the common good. That's what sovereign groups usually do. And no matter what good ideas they come up with, people are inclined to kick up. I mean, how come we are not talking to the counselling group and getting their thoughts about this afternoon?"

At an affective level, the answer to that question was easy. It seemed a horrible idea to waste group time traipsing over to the stables to talk to those kindly dimwits. One of the few pauses in this intense morning came here. Recording it, I marvel at how completely Manfred had disappeared from my awareness, and I think other people's. This seemed another example of a proper use of power. Manfred's sick, neurotic way of handling the world had re-surfaced in those last acts of departure. It would have been easy for us to respond by backbiting, by a have-over that would have been less an assimilation, than a reinforcement of bad feelings against someone to whom the group had given a great deal, and who had for a time given back with such riches and depth.

This aside is important to me. I see now the possibility that I am describing one of the curses of female observation. I saw the prince inside the frog, and wanted to pit all my strength to releasing him. I am guessing that something of the same is going on for Grace, when she looks at Pierre. Only he is more of a toad than a frog, at times. Perhaps it is more important for me to notice the princess in me and work to let her out. Somehow this connects to the meeting this afternoon.

I had put only a forty-five minute tape into the machine, and did not notice when it needed to be reversed, so again I have to rely on memory for the rest of this report.

Chuck was one of the people who was literally on his feet straight after Grace had talked about approaching the other group. He wanted to get over there and talk. But he dropped like a felled ox when Orminda said that we needed to decide how to make that approach, before rushing in. Sappho pulled a face and murmured about manipulation. Orminda said something that struck me very much, about the contact between groups needing to happen at an aware level. She compared what we were doing to the pre-contact phase of gestalt formation. Grace opened Ed Nevis's book (Nevis 1987) and said it had a picture of Chuck in it. It was a diagram of energy arousal and discharge, with the suggestion that there is a progressive quitting of the ground, as energy gets higher. Chuck nodded ruefully, and entered the discussion of tactics. I doubt if any of us had ever sat down before to plot an approach collaboratively in this way.

Going over en masse was the first idea, I do not remember from whom. Sohan said that we might look like an army knocking at the door, and the rest of us could imagine the defensiveness we might feel if the whole mass of counsellors came to us like that. Gradually we re-invented the idea of an ambassador or emissary. There was no trouble about granting full powers to this role. There was more trouble filling it. The competitiveness which is a feature among us seemed back again. Certainly I noticed a hope lying secret in me, that I should be called on. But my name was not mentioned. Grace offered herself, saying that pinko sentiments would keep the counsellors from being nasty to her. This seemed shrewd, but did not rouse enthusiasm. After various lackadaisical—by which I am sure I mean blocked-energy—suggestions, Pierre proposed Orminda, and we all agreed. She was in this shimmering, capable mode this morning. Her Irishness would register with some of the Irish nuns. There were all sorts of reasons. Yet I could not bring myself to look at Grace as we discussed when Orminda was to go over. Monarchy had risen again from the olden times of the beginning of the week. And this time Orminda, not Grace, seemed the queen.

While we had a very late coffee, Orminda drafted a letter, that we emended to the following version. She gave it to Maurice as he walked by. So in the end that was the full extent of her ambassadorship.

> *Dear Counselling Group,*
>
> *We have spent the morning brooding about the community meeting we shall be having this afternoon with you and the new Ecology Group. We are struck at how difficult we were in the first meeting this week, and are grateful for your patience in dealing with us. Now that we have thought through how helpful such meetings can be, we wonder whether you would join us for a pre-meeting, straight after lunch if that suits you. To cope with the large numbers who will be at the Community Meeting, it may be that we could work out a new structure.*
>
> *If you are interested, perhaps you would like to come over to the stream for coffee at one-thirty. Or we can come over to the stable block if you prefer.*

We all signed. Pierre said firmly that we were still hostile to them, and they were still hostile to us, as the new group would be hostile to all. Birde chided his determinist attitude, and said she had a different presentiment.

Sappho complained that our last full afternoon was going to be all work and interruption. I know I was regretting the loss of quiet time for being in this other world of flowers and terraces, leaded windows, massive oak stairs and fine rooms built for many to live together. My tall London house with its childless bedrooms now seems horrible by comparison, with its views of blank walls. Pierre commented these confessions as evidence of our hostility. I agreed.

Grace said, "It's a weakness of your method, to comment on hostility to the point where you provoke it. Then people are muddled. They can say you started it. And a weakness of Gestalt, specially in groups, can be to do a management job which avoids much hostility being felt, and certainly makes intra-group expression of it unlikely early on. For less biassed group development, you need to allow in good feelings, and we need to allow in bad feelings, in the initial stages. And I know that is a simplistic description. But it's true enough, if you want to hear me."

"And this afternoon we can perhaps explore these possibilities, at inter-group level," said Pierre. I felt a pang of relief, and realised that I had been braced for a defensive reaction from him. This was not the very last moment of the session. But it feels a right one to end on. It picks up the solidarity between us, which I connect to the threat of meeting the other groups. United we stand. Divided we may fall. I notice that I am scared.

Jan's comment

> Human beings always live in groups. Groups in turn cannot be understood except in relation to other groups and in the context of the conditions in which they live. We cannot isolate biological, social, cultural and economic factors, except by special abstraction. Mental life is the expression of all these forces, looked at horizontally, as it were, in the strictly present reality, and vertically, in relation to past inheritance. (Foulkes 1975)

This morning's meeting is an illustration of the lines quoted here. You are seeing a wider gestalt. You are grappling with the actuality of inter-group contact, and with sudden insights about tradition and acculturation. I am fascinated that this has been the progression from the pretty torrid sexuality of some recent sessions. In place of the feudal or tribal responses you had brought to the first inter-group exercise, you now accept belonging to your group and belonging to the historic, person-interchangeable group of this conference centre.

There is a doubt implicit in some of your comments, about whether the inter-group preoccupation is an avoidance of the centaur at home, below the table. Certainly the priorities have changed. From intense involvement with the two-person system, there is a compensating shift to the largest available system, one made up of almost fifty people. As the eyes rest from reading by looking at the view through the window, perhaps the minds of most of you in the group require a wider space and vision after days of close-focus and cluster.

Another idea is with me too, as I remember John Bowlby's

(1988) theory that, to be healthy, we all need a limited number of deep attachments, which are likely to start with pairing with our mothers. That suggests to me that we all have a capacity for intense belonging, which we can use in many ways. We can deny it, or experience it appropriately, which is to say, in a few places, or, from many needs or causes, overuse it dysfunctionally, as deprived children are variously observed to do. The need to belong, coupled with the old Law of Praegnanz, can result in crazy loyalties in most people, as most of you acknowledged round the time of the first meeting with the counselling group. Now you are moving into a new awareness of contact and connection, and of multiple boundaries which preclude you sticking with a Not In My Back Yard attitude to nearby groups.

Evolution as an aware process

The hypothesis was put forward in Chapter 10 that the life of a group is likely to be an allegory connected to the life of its individual members. On the next magnification, the co-creation of the intergroup contact boundary may have some of those same recapitulatory elements. But now an economy is evident. Eight people working in co-operation can learn faster than one person alone, just as eight people seemed able to work through mourning faster than one might have done alone. So the fore-contact processes of arousal, then finding what to do, become part of a spoken rather than an interior dialogue. You seem to have grown up fast, from street gang, to being easily respectful of the out-group and your interconnectedness.

If a group is to function for the enhancement of its members, they must have healthy intra-group contacts. Even these will not stay healthy unless there are cross-boundary contacts too. If intergroup systems are to flourish, the same obtains. It is likely that unless the sequence from personal, through group, to inter-group is worked through sufficiently, unaware frustration will be vented dramatically between the groups.

What is happening among you is what I guess needs to happen in every social system. Rather than accept the gloomy notions of Le Bon and McDougall (Freud 1921) of a loss of judgement and individuation in group membership, you are allowing awareness and judgement into the field. And that is where we have got to as a species. We are learning about our genes, and equipping ourselves to intervene biologically to modify ourselves in ways that may be outrageous or beneficent. And in just the same way, as we learn about our likely responses in groups, we can change them as we will. I guess in time these acquired characteristics will turn into an inheritance, both within each of us, and through the enduring social structures we invent to contain succeeding generations. There is so much to be done, my children.

References

Bowlby J. (1988) *A Secure Base*. London: Routledge.
Brown D. (1978) Toward a theory of power and intergroup relations. In: C. Cooper and C. Alderfer (Eds), *Advances in Experiential Social Processes*. Chichester: John Wiley.
Erikson E.H. (1964) *Childhood and Society*. New York: W.W. Norton.
Foulkes S. (1971) Access to unconscious processes in the group-analytic group, *Group Analysis* 4.
Foulkes S. (1975) Problems of the large group. In: L. Kreeger (Ed.), *The Large Group*. London: Maresfield Reprints.
Freud S. (1921) *Group Psychology and the Analysis of the Ego*. Harmondsworth: Penguin, 1991.
Gustafson J. and Cooper L. (1989) *The Modern Contest*. New York: W. W. Norton.
Jung C. (1959) Man and his symbols. In: W. McGuire (Ed.), *The Collected Works of C.G. Jung*. London: Routledge and Kegan Paul.
Knopf D. (1991) *Gestalt in Education*. Paper presented at Fifth Annual Conference of the Gestalt Association of the United Kingdom, Scotland.
Nevis E. (1987) *Organizational Consulting. A Gestalt Approach*. New York: Gardner Press, p. 26
Perls F., Hefferline R. and Goodman P. (1951) *Gestalt Therapy*, Vol. 2. New York: Dell.
Polster E. (1987) *Every Person's Life is Worth a Novel*. New York: Norton and Co.
Turquet P. (1975) Threats to identity in the large group. In: L. Kreeger (Ed.), *The Large* Group.
> Turquet uses the term *singleton* to describe this sense of unconnectedness that comes to many people in large groups.

Chapter 12

Thursday afternoon: Nodal points and self-regulation

Jan writes: The last movement of the symphony is under way by now. Most of the themes of the week are touched on in this account. How extraordinary that the group stays so figural for Orminda that she has been the scribe, when she sounds like one of the people most passionately involved in a sub-set of the group.

I was amazed that Orminda is so parenthetic, so by-the-way in reporting that Sappho and Chuck ignore the inter-group event, and pursue their non-Platonic private one. This would likely have resulted in trouble earlier in the week. But mellowness has supervened. Either the end is not to be spoiled, or people calculate that they can store their frustration for the one remaining day of the group. I will not discount that as a possible valency.

Your talk here, as reported, is a justification of experiential learning. New perceptions seem born as you speak, directly from what you have lived and are living through together. You accept, with your gut, or third eye, or with whatever integrative faculty one takes in the whole perception, that at times you feel like you are behaving as instruments of the group. The vectors in the field have quietly formed and influenced, and curious exchanges of task and behaviour appear, to some of you, to have resulted.

It is easy to suppose from the report that the majority of you are in the altered state of awareness that follows on continuous social stimulus in a sufficiently trusting group. But your feet are on the ground. This is not the Group Illusion (Anzieu 1975). This seems to me like final contact, a precious and fleeting time when the boundaries between your minds are so open that you are released into a mode where you see afresh and invent, are original, and function on love with less and less fear (Zinker 1977). The parting from all this may be hard, I register parentally. You are struggling with the implicit idea that much of what is happening is to do with the structure and process, and not with mere individual whim. The Gestaltists among you may be facing the possibility that even a simple idea like self-responsibilty is more intricately complex than it may have seemed before. And the attractions between you have become strong. You matter.

Orminda's account

When I said at the end of the morning that I'd write up this next session, I had the idea of it being a short one, what with the swimming and the big group meeting and maybe getting ready for some kind of a shindig tonight. And here I am writing up the lot. And doing it at twelve o'clock at night, sitting just outside the big oak door, drowning in honeysuckle, and watching a moon as big as a barrel go sailing across the clear sky. I'd call it a night for romance, if I wasn't communing with an exercise book and a biro.

Grace and Annie and Pierre and Sohan are sitting on the lawn by the pond. All the others are away to bed so far as I know. So it needs to be said that I shall stop writing if Pierre comes by here. And there's a real luxury in seeing him, being in earshot, and thinking he looks more social and easy than I have seen him. Non-possessive love. Limited by a kind of a yearning too. They have some paper in front of them, so maybe they are also writing up the group.

The last night. It's like being a child again, fighting fate, bargaining for one more look, one more bit of talk, before my Dad went off again across the water. I'm wrung out in my gut when I stop to notice, ready to sob, promising God whatever last little bit of a treat he wants so long as I can be in those arms again.

Life came and picked us up and ran with us from two o'clock this afternoon, when the counsellors brought their poor old floral skirts across here for our pre-meeting. And for the thousandth time I

Nodal points and self-regulation 161

made the discovery that The Others, The Outsiders, were devil and all the same as the insiders, as us. Except in this case that a couple of the nuns had been studying The Large Group, for use in their apostolic, and to help their own communities run better. So they were not the same as us, they were altogether better.

We kind of started the meeting being the gracious and forbearing hosts, handing out coffee and big smiles. Finding that we had experts among us wiped the smiles off our competitive faces. Annie, of all people, began to talk fast, explaining that we had our own theories and methods in The Large Group, but would be delighted to know theirs. Exclamation marks. That statement verged on the vainglorious, did it not? But the rest of us sat there and colluded silently with this defensive codswallop. I did not meet anyone's eyes, for fear of laughing, or feeling shame.

But what a power struggle! We had had this long talk all morning about the pitfalls, and here we were with our spades, digging great traps for ourselves and then merrily hurling ourselves in them. We had certainly avoided the sense of being isolates without identity in this invasion. Instead we were the besieged village, using subterfuge where we had no real weaponry or threats to offer to the enemy. Feudalism had sprung out of the wainscot of our anarchistic panelling.

I have never been hypnotised, but they tell me you stay aware: you just seem to decide to do what the suggester asks, even though you can still rationalise about it. That was me at that moment. I knew all that I have just written. Yet somehow or other I just happened, and the rest of us just happened, to go along with Annie's monstrous version of our expertise. Freud (1921) talks about hypnosis, then about love as the cohesive force in groups. Yes, a family loyalty sort of love was what I experienced.

And the counsellors came out shining. They never challenged us, or asked us to put our theories out for inspection. They did what we had said we would, and displayed their own concerns and vulnerabilities about the afternoon meeting. That was the way to reach us. Skilled workers called to the buried skilled workers in us. They did their Rogerian (Rogers 1973) thing, and asked us about the structure we had hinted at in our letter.

Grace pitched her voice right, just hesitant enough, and described our two, four, eight idea, and the rationale of it. From then on, all went as merry as a... That phrase upsets me. I stopped myself writing, so must write the resistance, to melt it, as Perls describes in Volume Two (Perls, Hefferline and Goodman 1951).

I can look back and say I have turned from a glacier to a river while I have been here. I flow again. And instead of that rigid unending pent-up pain inside myself, I'm maybe disastrously open, hoovering up new feelings and excitements everywhere I look. So in my head I tell myself that maybe I want Pierre so much because he is the dominant male in the herd. And because he is hard to get. I believe Sohan and Chuck. I could have had a decorous, subtle, deep and wistful liaison with Sohan, for the asking. With Chuck I could have had the physical passion I had forgotten I wanted, but that I tremble for now. I could have had it without much complication. So I go for the Oedipal non-solution, with Grace cast as mother.

Or is that just a cynical dismissal of a real recognition of my other half, my pair? Or am I just dazzled by the difference in his learning from mine? And when I have added some psychodynamic insights to my social science; when he is not the group prize; when I am not the Queen of the May any more, will my passion wither?

All these are the careful thoughts in my head. Then I sneak a look down towards where he is sitting by the pond, and they do not match the jolt like an electric shock as I scribbled towards the word Marriage, and found it so painful to write. I want to spend my life with him. I trust him and respect him and love his skinny body.

And much of what I love him for will stand in the way of his walking out on his sick wife.

Well, that is better out than in. And I hope he reads it, so there.

Back to the others. Pierre said to me as we walked over later to the whole community meeting, that task had finally tuned out affect, in that pre-meeting. I said it was more that the feeling—affect as he calls it—had supported the task (Palmer 1989). A sort of warmth came in, as we found the counsellors on our side. They found a way to save Annie's (which is to say our group's) face, and still move beyond pretence. I think we all saw that, and respected them for it. They lit a little good-deed candle in a naughty world.

Maybe twenty of the ecology group were assembled when we went into the barn. They had put up a lot of their educative posters,

Nodal points and self-regulation

like so many dogs marking their lamp-post, I thought, before maturity reassembled itself inside me. They seemed to have no resentments about what was in our minds a perilous attempt at take-over by the joint invaders. Grace and Maurice from the other group led off, suggesting the two-four-eight as a way of generating our needs of the meeting. One of them said she would like to know first how long we would meet for. We settled on an hour. Intellectually, I recognised that the ecology group had entered the ownership of the afternoon by this operation. And I could quieten a momentary peevishness that one of them had interrupted Grace.

I could almost say it all went too swimmingly. The pairs were all cross-group, and sat talking and smiling for their five minutes with what seemed total ease. The fours looked earnest and involved as they wrote headlines on their papers. There were finally forty-nine of us altogether, as some of their members came in in dribs and drabs over the first ten minutes. This is not the place, and it certainly is not the time of night, for me to go in detail into the lists that emerged from the sixteen stages of the exercise. The time was up by now. But they called for, and we accepted, a half-hour extension. We were all excited at the overlaps between what we were all wanting, and the understanding of how differently we had formed our needs, in the light of each other's.

I know I had gone to that meeting preoccupied with the process of it, with the how. And pulsing through me too was this excitement about the historical accretion or acculturation possible in this Conference Centre. And I did not let go of that, either. The counselling group seemed to put in more content-loaded stuff, like wanting to promote understanding between people, and offer their knowledge of what they called listening techniques. The ecology people were also into offering. The word "environment" came up a lot on their lists. I wish we could let them take over that word, and find a different one in Gestalt to describe the Other, the Outside. I hope Daniel Stern's notion of intersubjectivity gets hauled into Gestalt soon (Stern 1985). The post-Freudians have done as cackhandedly, with that terrible phrase "object relations". Relations means sexual relations, which means mortal sin, where I come from. Object looks like a verb, so I start thinking, O, they object to having relations. Other people are other people, don't you know? Calling them objects shows more respect for grammatical forms than for human souls.

We need a unifying vocabulary between all these disciplines. If we had that, we might stumble on a unifying theory. Which is what we all started to get excited about at this community meeting.

The ecologists asked on their lists for more expertise in running meetings and groups. They said they were worse at human relations than at environmental systems. So the ecology group gave us a confession of ignorance and a wish for our knowledge. We turned reciprocal, and spoke of our limited knowledge of ozone layers, greenhouse effect, and whether nuclear reactors are bad or good. And we were just raring to give them all the insight we could about group process. The half-hour passed, and still we sat there, sweating with enthusiasm and concentration. At a little after five we broke, with promises all round to put something on paper to give each other. One of the nuns suggested that we have a whip round and buy a box-file for the Centre, in which any bits of writing of this kind could be left. Didn't we all love ourselves? Synergy had struck, as we all went in for handshaking and the exchanging of addresses before departing for our separate teas.

There's a story in Machiavelli about Philomenon, who was a good general because he did nothing but rehearse battle strategies with his chums whenever they went for a walk in the country. What a bore. But there was something of the old fellow about our group. We had thought into, through and out the other side of that big meeting before we went into the barn to be present at it. Edgar Snow (1970) tells the same kind of a thing about Chairman Mao. On the Long March, he could always tell when there was going to be a big meeting, because of all the little pre-meetings Mao went in for. That's a different way of doing things, and maybe a more manipulative one. But Mother of God, a big meeting is a terrible wild creature if you have not thought beforehand what titbits you'll carry along for it to eat, and what kind of a net you have ready if it starts to play the devil with you.

What I entirely forgot to say was that Sappho and Chuck did not put in an appearance at the community meeting. They kind of melted away just before it. So there were six of us only in all that throng. But a strong presence, and one I was proud of. We all spoke up at different moments, and all to the point. Or is this just my group pride? At least it's my group understanding. We know so much about each other in this group now. Eighteen hours a day for four days, bad times and good. So when one of us speaks, I feel such a complication of love, and such a complex impression of the special meaning of them saying those words at this moment, and such a yearning for them to be received right.

Why don't I live in a group of people? The horror of the living alone I have been in these last months is grotesque to me now. And that little dark house is standing shut, waiting to ravage me again, in only a day and a half. Which reminds me, I have no idea where I shall stay tomorrow night before going off for my plane on Saturday.

We all went for a swim before our tea. Birde has a Scandinavian way of tearing her clothes off with no apparent self-consciousness. The rest of us did the same, with Pierre, seen in the very outermost corner of my peripheral vision, almost dying of embarrassment, I'll swear, before he turned his back and slipped his knickers down and then was into the water before I could fairly see whether he was a centaur or a merman or a well-hung brute of a fellow.

The being together was so important. It reminded me of that clanning there can be round the time of a funeral. I'm in mourning already for our end, I know it. Annie's jokes, Grace's strange changes of expression all in a moment, from comedy to tragedy, as her wide mouth turns up or down, quite out of her awareness; Pierre's hands; Sohan's earnest timid voice; Pierre's half-profile and a kind of turn of his neck he has; Birde's way of licking her lips when she disapproves; Pierre.

I think I was the one tonight to cajole us from the table, or try to. Again I had the fear that was there in the morning, of us slithering our avoidant way into disintegration.

I've been aware that our love-affair
Was too hot not to cool down.

I don't want us disappearing into the sunset on a raft of platitudes. It was not just one of those things. Yet, as Pierre would point out, that is the song that comes into my mind.

Here's hoping that we'll meet again
It was great fun,
But it was just one of those things.

Chuck and Sappho had evidently been on a trip to the moon on gossamer wings. I felt envy. And resentment. I said so. Grace did her Gestalt thing and made the Perlsian connection between resentment and appreciation. She used the word "value" where I'm used to "appreciation". I prefer her word; it belongs on this side of the Atlantic. From that we got into a whole long examination of how that flight into the pair had brought home to us the theory.

"Also," said Birde, "they express directly that little wish I had to be all the afternoon swimming."

"Wow," said Chuck, "so being in a group is one way of achieving omnipresence. In the hospital I'm always telling the nurses I didn't take the course yet."

"Excuse me, what course?" asked Sohan.

"The omnipresence course. But a group can do several things at the same time, instead of just thinking about them."

"And it's a function of strength of personality, as to which part of the group does which bit of the action," Annie added.

"Is it what you call strength of personality, or just where each person has got to in her life at that time—the achieved self?" Grace asked, thinking as she spoke, and speaking slow. Pierre came right back in the same tone, or as near it as he can ever get to being like another human being:

"This expresses my thought. I make an association between Sappho's not being with us, and her position in her family, also with her recent break with her lover in Athens. To go off with Chuck might for you, Sappho, have been at once the youngest child's rebelliousness, the quest for the lover, and the gratification of the swimming need that was in the group."

Grace had fetched Kreeger's *The Large Group* while we were talking, and now read out a piece. She had taken over one of Manfred's jobs, I thought. It was uncanny. She sounded excited.

"Psychoanalysis, sociology and gestalt psychology all contributed to the particular blend of theory that led Foulkes to evolve his concepts of the individual as a nodal point in a network of relationships, and to conceive of illness..."

She interrupted herself to explain that she was thinking of much more of our behaviour than just illness, then read on: *...as a disturbance in this network that manifests itself in and through the predisposed individual. The logical extension from this is the treatment of the network rather than treatment of the individual.*

Nodal points and self-regulation 167

"I bet that is not really a new idea to most of us, though it is so clearly expressed. It's just that I am living it at the moment, seeing how each thing we do seems a sort of pressing up to the surface of the most predisposed person. And we've all done the pressing, one way or another."

We took time chewing through this idea, which was newer, to me at least, than Grace had suggested. Annie had been making faces, and said, "Sappho and Chuck didn't gratify my swimming need. They did that for them, maybe, but not for me."

"So maybe the individual learning, the bit in this for you, is to find how you suppress your swimming need, and let Sappho instead of you be the most predisposed thingummy." Annie nodded, and again I had that strange disorienting sense of a new idea rearranging everything in my mind, like a new instruction on the word-processor which sends the whole machine into a minute of buzzing withdrawal. After that everything on the screen looks different.

Chuck answered Grace as if Annie had not spoken: "That's as neat a description of an over-determined piece of behaviour as I could find. And for me, the going off had more to do with that dread of my uncle, and the whole threatening older generation power structure when I was a kid. At work I turn into one of the bosses in order to survive in big meetings. Here I fled, the way I used to with my sister."

"And did you treat me as you treated your sister?" asked Sappho, in a provocative voice. Chuck showed more awareness than she seemed to, or at least, more sensitivity to the group, by glancing round and saying, "I might as well tell you, we didn't have one of those Platonic afternoons."

There was a two-beat silence, then Sohan had to have the Platonic reference explained to him. He said, "I think Pierre's and Grace's idea is also in this. But like Annie, I think too that it is not satisfactory to me to have others do my making love." There was a lot of smiling and nodding. He added, "I have felt such strong physical needs that I have relieved them with my hand, in a way that has not happened since my marriage."

I was in a mortal agony that other people would start to make sexual confessions. I couldn't. I wouldn't. So, thinking of the metaphor we were using, it seemed that the wish for inhibition won out just here. Chuck took Sohan's hand and squeezed it, so he was kind of acknowledged. Then we dropped into a brooding silence for a minute or two, till I said out some of what I have just written. People looked ready to move subjects, and Annie introduced one, by going back to her joke about letting another part of the group express something, rather than do it yourself. Already she seems fully back in the group, in a way I thought might not happen, when I saw her looking so devastated, so old, to be truthful, at the beginning of today. I thought she had gone into a depression that would sink her into a silent withdrawal from the last days of the group. So maybe we did do an accelerated piece of shared mourning, as we talked of.

She referred to the wake for Manfred, as a task that needed the whole group. Then she talked about specialism, about the ablest at particular tasks taking them over, so that the whole group worked more effectively than one individual.

"It's back to the idea of Orminda as leader, or expresser, of something about survival from utter cruelty." I interrupted to remind her of Sohan's story, which he has told to a few of us, but not mentioned in the formal group sessions. She added him, then said, "And Sohan has stood for a sort of simplicity and openness to learning, that gradually we took on, but that has stayed his specialty. Sappho has been our passion in contact, in approach."

"Even invasion, I think," said Sappho, and people laughed, relieved that she was not going to be cross.

"Pierre is the holder of honour and learning and inhibition."

"That makes me the bad guy," said Chuck, not joking at all. "I don't know that I want to carry looseness and lust for the group."

"In a confluent group, I think we could easily have become imitators of Grace or of Pierre in particular. They are two models of group expertise and insight," Annie continued. "But I feel more myself than before I arrived, not more like them. I've learned from everyone. Everyone. And to the discerning eye, threads of all of you will show in the weaving of the rest of my life."

"Turquet added a fourth basic assumption to Bion's theory," said Pierre. "He called it 'fusion', a kind of loss of individuality in order to express group membership. Perhaps the Gestalt word 'confluence' allows for more motivations behind the behaviour. I am not sure if we are confluent, or if we are more clearly differentiated after our days together. Time will perhaps tell."

"I cannot bear these valedictions," said Sappho. "We are not dead yet."

"So why don't we get up and dance," said Pierre, not as a question, but as a little tease. And maybe as a route to touching me, for that is what happened when we finally did dance later on. He held me in a smoochy nightclub body-to-body way, and I would not talk. Me so gabby and with my mouth by his ear, and needing nothing but the presence of him, without these redundant accompaniments of speech.

But before that there was protest that we must consider the Last Day. Most pressingly, the ecology group had asked if we would join them in the morning, to teach them something about group process. Did we want to use our time that way? There was nothing easy about the decision. I had certainly not made my mind up beforehand. Neither did anyone else seem to have done. But we came out with a yes. The counselling group have left. So it will be the eight of us to nearly thirty of them, with all the feelings that involves. We decided to plan nothing until possibly at breakfast, except that, come what may, we would have our last afternoon in our own group.

"We are withdrawing in some ways," said Grace, "or I am. We keep saying that we are not making our disclosures so carefully at the beginning of sessions now. And for me that is to do with not wanting to open wounds I can't heal before I leave. I'm so grateful to the people who keep open in different ways. I am, in some ways. But I doubt if I am the only one making some judgements about lauching into some whole new area of uncharted embarrrassment or pain in myself, at this stage. So a worst fantasy comes up, of us turning out to be a bit flat or silent tomorrow morning.

My biggest excitement right now is about how we define ourselves as a group. When we're like this, I feel the preciousness to me, the specialness of every one of you. The most human humans. The angels on earth. Something as exaggerated as that. Then when we meet the others, I fancy a membrane, maybe in a different colour, that delineates us, separates us from them, and is also the place of contact, of meeting them."

"Being the pedagogues to the ecology group preserves and strengthens this surrounding membrane," said Pierre, half interrogative, so I am not sure whether to write a question mark. Once more he had answered straight back to something Grace said. A form of polygamy, I thought to myself. Grace is number-one wife, who shares the head-of-family position. I am number-two wife, perhaps.

If he allowed himself a concubine, I think I would be her. No, I do not like this notion of polygamy, with its male-centredness. Polyandry too, please. We are all proactive in these multiple pairings. And we can be safe in them, as we are all witnesses to the extent and kind of involvement we have. That is the weird sense of freedom here, that I am known to everyone in such intimate ways, and still accepted.

Strangely, I do not think Pierre would have allowed his feeling for me even to come to consciousness, if he had not been surrounded by the group. Conversely, maybe Sappho would not have needed to invade Chuck—for I'll bet you a shirehorse to a maggot that that was the way round of things between them. She would not have needed to do that if she had not been reacting to the competitition in the group, and to that transferential stuff she talked about earlier.

A powerful configuration, a group.

Pierre has stood, and taken a step backwards away from the others. He looked this way for a moment.

Jan's comment

Implicit in this account is the experience of final contact, in Perls' sense. The group has apparently at many moments become properly confluent within itself. It functions effectively, without the intrusion of the inter-personal, in such moments as the meeting with the big group, when Chuck and Sappho are not even there, and yet the group is not disrupted. A less healthy confluence shows when Annie boasts unchecked to the counsellors. Orminda speaks of trance in this context. In the first instance, an overt goal of the group was dealt with in a way that met the ambition of each member, so far as we can tell. In the second, a remaining bit of the denied wish for supremacy came out of the unlikely nodal point, Annie. This example is a reminder that more than the ego, the overt, the accepted, can surge into inter-group relations, unless there is more education about them than our group has had. The counsellors do better. So in this instance, a one-sided dialogic approach was enough to nudge you lot back into the same mode.

Final contact

Final contact is the consummate moment of merging, when figure and ground have reversed, perceptually, or, put another way, the contact-boundary itself is figural. A group of soldiers working as a team in the midst of a battle is a group example: loading and firing, aiming, protecting, changing ground—all these occur at times in a way that is the very opposite of Each Man For Himself. This temporary merging is an extraordinarily important group phenomenon. It tends to be commented on pejoratively at social level, if at all (Lifton 1986). Yet it looks as if members of groups are seeking this state, with energy, from early in the group life. Communitas is the inchoate hope (Goodman 1947). Rather than a pathological gratification or a group illusion, it is arguable that the phenomenon has the potential for personal transcendence and altruism. How it manifests is a function, not of process alone, but of process on the background of content.

I wish I knew whether the synergy of this time is just to do with a coincidence of need in most of you, to make an honest investigation of group process, and so end up with your personal working hypotheses and theory. I need to remind myself and you that you are fulfilling most exquisitely my ambition for the group. Does some of the blessed, the radiant feeling that is around, relate to being good children? One small advantage of being an absent leader, I guess, is that you never get to see the holes in my socks, and my Achilles' heel through them. I can remain a bit of an ideal figure, for whom the reports are still prepared, even in such poignant circumstances as Orminda's this summer midnight.

References

Anzieu D. (1975) *The Group and the Unconscious*. Trans. B. Kilborne. London: Routledge and Kegan Paul, 1984.

Foulkes S. and Anthony E. (1957) *Group Psychotherapy—The Psycho-Analytic Approach*. Harmondsworth: Penguin.

Freud S. (1921) *Group Psychology and the Analysis of the Ego*. Harmondsworth: Penguin, 1991.

Goodman P. (1947) *Communitas*. New York: Random House.

Lifton R. (1986) *The Nazi Doctors*. New York: Basic Books.

Palmer B. (1989).
> In a presentation at Goldsmith's College, Barry Palmer described a schema of the four ways a group can function: 1. The task is all, and affect is suppressed. 2. Affect is all, and the task is suppressed. 3. The mood supports the task. 4. The mood generates the task.

Perls F., Hefferline E. R. and Goodman P. (1951) *Gestalt Therapy. Excitement and Growth in the Human Personality*, Vol. 2. New York: Julian Press.

Pines M. (1975) Overview. In: L. Kreeger (Ed.), *The Large Group*. London: Maresfield Reprints.

Rogers C. (1973) *Carl Rogers on Encounter Groups*. Harmondsworth: Penguin.
> In this and other works on client-centred therapy, Rogers advocated starting where the client is. By this he meant, exploring the client's world rather than imposing your own prejudice on the meeting.

Snow E. (1970) *Red China Today*. Harmondsworth: Penguin.

Stern (1985) *The Interpersonal World of the Infant*. New York: Basic Books.

Zinker J. (1977) *Creative Processes in Gestalt Therapy*. New York: Brunner-Mazel.

Chapter 13

Friday morning: The group boundary

Jan writes: It has happened again. I pick up the typescript of this session, and find myself open-mouthed at who has written it. Maybe Pierre would reckon he was trying to sublimate some of the agitated energy which shows clearly in the opening paragraphs. He is another of you who appears to become more insightful when in erotic upheaval. The in-love state gets a pretty bad press in some quarters, being written off as euphoric and deluded. Just as communitas can lift a whole group, so I see the spin-off of generosity and wide vision that spreads out beyond an in-love pair, to affiliative relations, to the group. All that looks to me a healthy function of the cloud-nine phase. It may be there in Pierre as he writes.

One of the many themes which is discussed by the group here in a way novel for the speakers, is definition of the group by the outgroup or environment. This is a recapitulation of Perls' and Lewin's already quoted definition of the contact boundary. This is the creation by both the subject of the organism, the group here, and what is perceived beyond. The ecology group is making the contact boundary as much as the Manor group does. What is not explicit in this account is the sense of the power relation between the two. Yet it is crucial to what goes on.

Pierre's account

It is a madness that I write this. My physical state is quite deplorable. I eat almost not at all. For two nights I am without sleep.

But through last night, into many hours of quite subjective preoccupations, came many thoughts of this meeting between the groups. These I must record before proceeding.

I have considered the experience of group membership, and the cognitive processes by which this is created and maintained. The self-categorisation theory of J. C. Turner (1986) has been in my mind. He claims a certain depersonalisation whenever group membership is internalised. The member defines himself by a shared characteristic of the ingroup, or a difference with the outgroup, rather than by his purely personal attributes. As I write this phrase I acknowledge, today more than before in my life, that the purely personal is in itself a social construct.

O God, the purely personal, the id, the great surge of directed libido exists too, wells in my breast and in my gonads. Yet for part of the night I occupied myself with these speculations about the silent transactions each person in our group has made, in order to construe himself as one of the group. And in parenthesis I note that this nightwork is perhaps part of what Turner describes. I am corporate man for a brief time. It is an act of love towards that compelling fiction in my mind, the group itself, to lie awake and consider the origins of our cohesiveness. I am defining the group, and doing so in the face of this threatened meeting with the outgroup. Secretly, I form a skin around Us, to separate and preserve Us. This I am sure of. The sense of belonging is passionate and aware, and makes me suppose it is just as strong when repressed and unaware.

I would say that in our group we see ourselves first as students, even as clerks, as the monks of old. So it becomes important for us that we hold the vow of chastity, even in such personal turmoil as I suffer now. A part of being students is to reveal ourselves in a way that could be damaging if told in other contexts. So the chevalier joins the clerk in our group identity; there is a code of honour among us. Then there is this great sensitivity, required in our contemplation of the life Orminda has suffered, or Sohan for that matter. It has been reinforced in such episodes as the poetic farewell between Annie and Manfred. Such memories as these, I confess it, give me a sense of privilege, of being part of a completely special, a unique group.

I force myself to admit that I have observed such sentiments in myself and others on many occasions, at this stage of a group. The

The group boundary

common phenomenon is the definition of the group as apart, and probably superior. Yet never before have the feelings been so strong for me. I think my life changes dramatically in this time and after it. Or have I thought that also, in other places, in other groups?

So. Chastity wins. And that seems to me part of the depersonalisation process of which Turner speaks.

> ...the individual minds which enter into the structure of the group mind ... do not construct it; rather, as they come to reflective self-consciousness, they find themselves already part of the system, moulded by it, sharing in its activities, influenced by it at every moment in every thought and feeling and action... (McDougall 1921)

No. I sense myself in an intellectual agitation which is erotic in origin. Grace's face comes before my inner eye, with Orminda's beside it, and they reproach me for these thoughts, which speak of a helplessness of the collective. What about our Gestalt responsibility for self? they seem to ask me. I too strive for this awareness their doctrine so recommends, an awareness which allows me to see these formative forces as they impinge on me from the past and from the surrounding and intruding present. I do not any longer know if I hold my body away from Orminda's so-receptive and so-needy presence because I am a married member of the Catholic church, or because of my vows of abstention as a member of my professional association, or from a self-definition as one of these knight-students of this present group. Or does my fear of impotence or some other humiliation of intimacy keep me so high-principled? In other words, does the personal override the sense of group membership? How can I understand this forest as I stand in the twilight created by it?

To the morning. At breakfast there was much looking into each other's faces, much taking of hands for a moment, between eating and talking and making the last jokes about the toaster, the last morning pot of tea. All feel the loss that will come this very afternoon, as we take our bags and cases and direct ourselves to cars and taxis and trains and planes, far from each other. I do not know how I can tolerate the loss.

Also there was fragment upon fragment of comment which was

a definition of this group. I had strongly the sense of the skin of likeness we fabricate, and which we strengthen by talk of the difference of the Others, in this case the ecology group.

I remember Grace saying, almost with apology, "We're, I don't mean we're really a more profound group than them. But we've been thinking about deep issues, and we're by training concerned with the inner world, the less obvious." Implicit was it that the ecology group, concerned with the outer world, was somewhat less profound than us.

Sohan wanted us to make a list of what we would teach, in case we let the side down, as he said in his strange old-fashioned British idiom. Annie commented how important she was making it that we give a good account of ourselves to the other group, then saw the adversarial undertone of her anxiety. Orminda, suddenly like the Maid of Orleans, stood up, pale, and declared:

"We shall be invaders this morning, so the other group will have the terror that we are taking them over. But we are far fewer than them, so we shall have the terror of being taken over. We think we are better than them because we brood about the human spirit and the collective unconscious. We secretly fear they may be better than us because they are out there in the world trying to stop the planet being suffocated, tree by tree, factory by factory, car by car. If in our arrogance we hide this we betray ourselves and them."

As if she had not spoken, Sappho said, "I vote that we work with them from ten till twelve, and then come back here to ourselves, however hard they try to stop us." I pointed out how her statement reinforced the truth of what Orminda was saying. But Sappho said she did not really want to teach the others, anyway, so she was not interested. Now it was Birde who spoke quietly, suggesting that Sappho said loudly a little of what several of us might feel. She admitted her own resistance to the meeting, as well as interest in it. She feared it might be an avoidance of the end.

"All action is avoidance," said Grace. "Another figure is that we are working directly at the whole point of this week—at learning and passing on skill in making groups work for their purposes."

"That is our immortality," said Annie, clearing the table. "And how are we going to plan it?" All in the midst of loading the dishwasher and wiping surfaces, the women went on with what

The group boundary

was certainly a most productive conversation. But it is beyond me to think in one topic while my body is engaged with another. Before my wife's illness I remember the same quality in her, and recall my intolerance of it.

But from this few minutes we made a plan that Grace should arrive alone two minutes early. She quoted research by someone called Wilder (1981), about individuation, by which I think he meant meeting by ones, reducing or blurring group boundaries. The rest of us were to arrive all together about five minutes later. In this way she could direct the others to notice the different emotions aroused by the two entries. After that we might encourage a more democratic conduct of the morning.

And so it was. I remembered again Lorenz's observation about sensitive dependence on initial conditions in non-linear systems (Gleick 1988). The initial conditions partially existed in the common choice of this place for our two groups to meet. They existed also in our first meeting yesterday. But this morning is a unit in itself, whose initial conditions likewise merit respect and attention.

When the party of us minus Grace entered the lion's den, the lions were seated on the ground at the feet of Grace, with some quite unspeakable formless New Age music being played on a tape. There was some comment on my expression, I recall. Inwardly I criticised Grace for not making a strong interpretive comment, or process comment as she no doubt prefers to say. But she did well. Only at the end of the morning did she invite people to recall our entrance. By then they were habituated to the idea that it is scientific, not immoral, in such a gathering as we were, to report accurately on their emotionality.

Sappho and Chuck began to dance to this droning tape when they came in, and in this they were joined by a number of young men in long parti-coloured shorts of hideous aspect, which seemed fabricated from parts of curtains. My eyes went to the windows; however, they were draped in more tasteful cloths than covered these gyrating pelvises before me. Sohan had spoken before we set out of how we should dress for the meeting. I had been adamant in refusing to adapt. Grace had mentioned an experiment by Worchel and others (1978) in which having red coats for one group made them less attractive to a white-coated group than another white-coated group.

I have great resistance to telling in detail the part of the morning spent with the ecology group, except to emphasise the great diplomacy and calm with which Grace and indeed all the women conducted our side. I force myself a little. For more than half an hour we talked in small groups, consisting of four of the ecology group and one of us. The numbers worked almost precisely. The ecology groups chose themselves into this configuration on the base of being partial strangers. This lack of acquaintance with each other turned out to be a major theme, which Orminda and Grace addressed when we had reformed into the large group. Sappho then suggested a sociogram for them, which immediately took the form of them clustering in four groups, before wandering more to the centre, then, with much ashamed laughter, running back to these four groups. It appears that the groups were regional. It astonishes me that on this small island people can consider for a moment that they come from different regions. However, between us, we uncovered many fears and resentments about power being kept in Oxfordshire, where this movement had started, and where indeed we are as I write. An agreement to have their next conference in Scotland was made in our presence, and there was recognition of the new sub-groupings that are forming which break regional demarcations.

In two hours we passed on a remarkable amount of insight. Orminda has at this moment looked over my shoulder and accused me of arrogance. I write again: We enabled the ecology group to make these insights. Now Orminda has walked on down the steps to the lawn, and I see why I write with such speed and impatience. I say again, we did a very fine organisational consultancy for this ecology group.

She is going to swim, and I shall go too. It is a last time. The sky is blue as in the Midi. This is time outside time.

Moments so small, as when she pushes her hair behind her ear, will fill the rest of my life.

In the same manner as I write this account, convulsing inwardly at every other moment with strong emotion towards Orminda, and towards the coming farewell to all these people to whom I now have such tenderness as I had forgotten I could endure, so was the last part of the morning, from twelve to one. We sat once more in our own group, in the library. Orminda had been too

The group boundary

much in the sun yesterday and wished to be inside. Also, there was about us a task-oriented feeling. On Blake's grid (Blake and Mouton 1964) I think all seemed to rate near nine:nine. Full attention to task, combined with full attention to people and affect.

I was aware of cohesiveness, and explained my thoughts to some extent, in terms of Cartwright and Zander (1968) and their strong emphasis on interdependence. Grace cited Lewin (1948) as antecedent in his description of the group as a dynamical whole. I admit that I was encouraged that more people than I had expected seemed to know what they were talking about. My intellectual arrogance operates specially towards the English, I notice, whom I consider in general a badly-educated nation. Yet I think it was Annie who countered Grace's reference to Lewin, saying that he alleged that the dynamical whole existed independent of similarities or differences, meaning interpersonal attraction, between group members. She considered that our group cohesiveness was more in line with the notion held by Festinger and others (1950), that similar values and views underpin good group formation.

At this point Sappho screamed and said that if we did not speak of ourselves, she would walk out. Chuck said immediately that if she behaved once more like an infant he would hit her. One week ago this would have been the beginning of a major Greek tragedy. Now she said quietly, "I try," and he took her hand. Birde too called for concrete reference to ourselves, and took Sappho's other hand for a second. I think of transactional analysis, with its description of interactions as analogies for physical strokes (Samuels 1971). These are often expressed directly now between us, as I described at breakfast. Words may or may not accompany them: but the meaning seems recognised and appreciated mutually. I greatly appreciate the value of this behaviour, but have personal difficulty in copying it. This is certainly a measure of how I sexualise contact, and indeed, spend much time imagining physical contact with one person in particular. My guilt seems ineradicable.

To an outsider this contact from Chuck might have seemed extraordinary, abusive, sexist. Between those two, in this context— and I emphasise, within the safe context of this group—this exchange carried quite other values. There was a subtext of eroticism and teasing which both well understood, as I think did all others.

Our communication has become at once so economical, and so charged with undertones and overtones that transmit without the barrier of hostility and mistrust.

Chuck said that Manfred perhaps supported the Lewinian view of the dynamic whole, in two ways. First, he had been seen as dissimilar, and yet there had been great and ultimately successful efforts to integrate him into the group. Conversely, the group had continued to function well since his departure; the whole is therefore seen to be a system not dependent on each member. I remembered the absence of Chuck and Sappho yesterday afternoon, but forbore to support Chuck with this other piece of evidence.

"And Jan is a cipher in all this to some of us. We have no idea whether he is similar or dissimilar; but he feels to me to be a member still, in some symbolic and godlike way," said Annie.

"He's not a member as far as I am concerned," said Sappho, "until he bothers to be here for me to have a smell of him."

I picked up on this statement, interpreting it as implying that her criterion for membership was interpersonal attraction, as in the Festinger theory, and Byrne (1971).

The process of the group at this time seemed dictated by its stage, but in a way I would not have foreseen. Rather than stay in the enjoyment of the rich affective life that has developed among us, we were using that affect to underpin as theoretical a discussion as we have had. In my case, however, I comprehend the possible pain-avoidance in my devotion to the theoretical. We sat forward in our chairs, speaking one on another, but slowly, often staring gravely at one another as our thoughts developed. Birde raised a most fascinating issue:

"Once more I think of the relation of the pair to the group. Please, is it that this group exists only to support these three pairs among us?"

"What three pairs?" asked Grace. Birde looked surprised and answered, "I think of Annie and the now-absent Manfred; Chuck and Sappho; Pierre and Orminda. And I think too of the *Sociology of Georg Simmel*, in which he tells that the pair is the basis of all social organisation."

"Adam and Eve are proof of that," said Sappho, adding, "I hoped that we had said every word that could be said about pairs. Subject finished."

The group boundary

"In this group are many other pairs," said Sohan, and Sappho made noises of protest.

"Sexual attraction pairs," said Birde, "are what I speak of, since interpersonal attraction was our subject." At this point I remarked that Grace and Sohan looked levelly at one another for a moment. I formed the strongest impression that they had become one of these sexual pairs, but not at the level only of attraction; rather of carnal fulfilment. As my impression also is that their races are often at enmity, I was the more surprised, and suddenly angry. I voiced my suspicion and Sohan said that it was without foundation, at least in the matter of enactment. He added, "Certainly I have great awareness of the sensuality of Grace."

"Without the influence of Pierre, we might have had a right little knocking shop going on here," said Orminda. The expression had to be explained to me. I see that she was in part lightening a difficult moment. I notice too that, like Sohan, I think I am a most humourless person. At the time I could only wonder at whether I was indeed the superego of the group. It seemed likely. How futile.

Annie spoke, and I choose to record what she said, rather than pursue my narcissistic thoughts.

"I used to supervise a nun. She told me that after she had applied to enter a nunnery, she fell madly in love with a young man. She went and told the Mother Superior, who told her to take time to make up her mind. Finally she decided to take orders, and the Mother said to her something like, *you saw you had too much love to direct all at one person*. I think this group has been one where we have often been responsive to a more collective feeling than just the pair. We have needed each other for the task we are doing. Berkowitz calls that 'interactive interdependence'. Liking each other, or rather, honouring, respecting each other, has developed from that. I think that's called Equity Theory (Berkowitz and Walster 1976)."

"We don't all like each other," said Sappho. "I think many of you do not much like me."

"You act at times as if we did not," said Birde, once more with an acuteness I forget she has. She added, "When you have interrupted other people I have hated you for moments. And I was envious that you enchanted Chuck. That is not about disliking you, but more, disliking myself for being this thin spinster."

"Every word that every person utters now has a charmed quality," said Annie. "I am in the in-love feeling at a collective level, and Pierre can take his friend Anzieu and jump in the lake about that. This consciousness is the touchstone. It will not last; but it makes the measure of health and right mindedness for me, that I shall not forget." We sat quiet, for she had said what I and I think all could recognise as their own experience. She had thought further with it. Interdependence became a word with poignancy and life. Without her I would not have given such value to my present anguished experience.

"Until now," said Grace, "I have had such trouble with Friedman's idea of the between. Contact of I and Thou, yes. But the creation of the between sounded redundant. Now I wonder if he meant this environment, this tribal rhythm we have here. Maybe some of what we are saying now, we might have said on other days, in other tones of voice. But we all give out words with a sort of care, and let them inside us slowly, with so much recognition of what is behind and around each last statement. The only image I can find for it is that our words are silver, and we place them on black velvet as we speak, now."

After nods, and some quiet, Birde said that she had during the week been preoccupied with the idea of contact, and now she was thinking of the contacts between groups.

"Orminda told me some theory yesterday, about the greater the difference between groups, the greater the sense of belonging, within each group (Buss and Portnoy 1967). Then at breakfast this morning, people spoke of how to dress for our meeting with the ecology group. Some of us even said we would dress to be like them. So I think of confluence. Did we try to deny the difference between us, and make a confluence, to make one group of the two? I think not, for at the same time we spoke often, as Pierre reminded us, of our differences. With our clothes we thought to pretend confluence. With our ideas we tried to make separation from the other group." Her words were given great attention by the Gestalt practitioners.

"Now I think of Detlef Knopf's summary of the four kinds of learning. They might hold for all scenes. I think the first was, when what is outside and what is inside were formerly experienced as one, differentiation between them is clarified, so that proper assimilation happens. Second was a strengthening of the boundaries to keep

The group boundary

out the not-mine, the not-ours. That was all our stuff at breakfast about being geniuses of the psyche and all that. Third came what he called completion, the assimilation of the interesting new. That's what we wanted to enable in the ecology group; and I think we did some of that in those conversations over at their place. The last sort of contact was just noticing the novel, enough to let it do what he calls excite the boundaries; that results in energy, perhaps to reject or contest or create differently, rather than to incorporate."

"That is so much for me to think about that I want you to write it down," said Annie.

"I think I managed completion. You are giving form to what I was stumbling to think," said Birde. Orminda said to Annie, "Pierre has written it already." She had not even glanced in my direction. Her peripheral vision is remarkable.

"Those four modes more or less tie up all the ways groups can make useful contact, don't they?" asked Chuck. "And in Gestalt language, the unhealthy meetings would be confluence rather than integration. Some idea of Small is Beautiful (Schumacher 1973) comes in here. Keeping a sense of small group membership seems like sanity, even in a large group. The ecology group turned out to be a collection of sub-groups. It's back to the old Gestalt flicker, the old Heraclitan flux, between different perceptions from moment to moment. I could join the ecology group in the common fate of realising that we are suffocating the planet, actively, at every minute that we don't do something to reverse that. But then I was a member of this group again, knowing that this morning's task was to let them see how to manage human small systems more effectively. Membership of this group was vital to me for that, both for a sense of identity and confidence, and for the data, the back-up of exercises and examples and what all."

"You're saying that if we had just used Knopf's fourth mode, contacting the novel to excite our boundaries, but not to incorporate, that would have been another kind of unhealthy meeting?"

"Mode two, the strengthening of the boundaries in the face of the other, would have been just as useless," said Birde.

"None of these modes are good or bad in themselves. They belong to different fields, different scenes," said Grace. "If the other group had been intent on persuading us to start a riot or something, we might have done very well to use modes two or four. Meaning is a function of background and foreground. See Perls and Padrewski, passim."

"I need to go over what we did do," said Birde. "First we sent..."

Sohan interrupted her: "Excuse me, I think first we made many preparations. Our meeting was not impulsive. And I am thinking that it is always thus. To meet one other person, I can perhaps let myself do, what do you say? flying by the seat of the pants. But for a meeting between group and group, much conferring is needed beforehand."

Birde nodded and continued, "You have reminded me that I could liken the meeting to the Gestalt cycle of experience. Even that I have adapted in my mind this week, seeing always two cycles, yours and mine, and noticing the way they meet or do not. First as you remind me we became aware of the other group and of ourselves as we are contrasted to them. We went through arousal, and the spinning of ideas of how to make our contact. Sending Grace first was almost a fore-contact, a diagnostic probe."

"When I saw her walk across the yard, I wanted to give her a white flag," said Sappho. "No, don't laugh at me. I felt the risk of sending her alone like a hostage."

"Yes," said Annie, "and there was also the symbolic trust, in exposing just one of us to the thirty of them. I am not laughing at your image, Sappho. I think you saw what at other times I might forget to notice, in the menace and fear around the outgroup."

"I've been struggling with Perls' first book this week (Perls 1947)," said Chuck. "He has all these eating images. I can fancy us letting ourselves be chewed and assimilated, in a little touch of symbolic cannibalism, when we went into those sub-groups of six people. Then we magically reconstituted into this group again. Jeez, I must watch it. I'll spook myself, verging on the mystical here. It wouldn't go down well where I come from."

"So the family and the cultural group enter your awareness for a second, to warn you not to lose your idiosyncracy, even in this..." I did not have the English word till Orminda found it for me. I meant to term this group a haven, which it has been in some ways. When first she said it, I heard it as Heaven. So I wish for a Heaven group. And I look with dread to the Hell I fear will follow it.

The point I had first wanted to make was the likeness between person to group, and group to group. The sense of identity with the small significant unit seeks to be maintained in the face of the

The group boundary

larger present configuration. So the person is forming and being formed by his reference or other salient group. And we have seen ourselves striving to form our skin as a group, and make an identity which will not merge with that of the outgroup. The work is vital for the preservation of benchmarks of meaning and value.

These Gestalt pictures in books, which demonstrate that the urns or the profiles, the old woman or the young, can only alternate as figures of perception, have their use; but it is limited. The interesting dynamic is between fields, for example the inner and the outer world. Perhaps the camera makes a good analogy here. We have the ability to make a dynamic of perception constantly between a wide view, and then a zoom, a close focus on a significant part of the field. The fixed stare, the wandering middle field gaze, the shortsighted peer at detail, are all distortions of perception. It is this dynamic, this constant reforming of data into new configurations, which is health and growth. I congratulate myself. I speak deliberately in terms of Gestalt. To do so is a gift to myself, and also a kind of bunch of roses picked by a clumsy boy to offer to the loved one. I do not any more know if this is one woman, or the group.

Jan's comment

There is an openness, a vulnerability, in Pierre's account, which is the strongest testimony to the quality of *final contact* which prevails now in the group. He goes on with the theme Orminda made figural in the last report. That's no surprise to any of us. He too is aware of that special *between* quality, that in this meeting allows more chewing-through dialogue about current experiences. So I shall let myself comment about the only thing I notice Pierre leaving out. I get the suspicion that *post-contact* is subtly coming up alongside final contact. Some of the material here is a re-working, a cud-chewing, of important happenings that have already been commented. So to my mind we are back with this notion touched on already in the Dialogue session, of the post-contact phase which leads to the completion of any gestalt. You really look like you are savouring and chewing, with more retrospective attention, before the gestalt of this group starts to fade down and dim in your awarenesses, in that healthy loss of interest which is the usual description of Gestalt post-contact and completion.

Post-contact has a subtle series of sub-phases within it, I reckon, and you may be in the first of them, the thorough chewing. In passing, I notice some of what you are not chewing over, at least as Pierre reports you. Your cohesiveness is not complete in time or membership. Manfred, for example, was a refuser of group norms for much of the time he was a group member. Chuck and Sappho failed to come to a meeting where they were expected. But overall, as the carefully written accounts of the sessions in themselves testify, there has been high respect for the group and its task.

Whether interdependence has led to mutual attraction, or the other way about; whether the life-stories of many members have led to the strong sexual charge in the group; whether pre-conditions of similarity between people led to cohesiveness, are subjects for surmise rather than conclusion.

A different explanation none of you offered perhaps merits a word here. Gestalt presents us with two concepts which can appear contradictory. One is the indivisibility of figure and field. Extrapolated, this approaches some of the Eastern philosophy of One, of I am That, of the unity of all. This can be seen as another way of saying that cohesiveness is the real or underlying state. Separateness is an illusion.

However, Gestalt also contains the idea that contact involves separateness. Translating these two ideas to this group, it could be said that, just before its dissolution, members can glimpse something as close to Oneness as is available to human consciousness. The conditions for this are clear. Most of them have been spelled out already. One that can be emphasised is the way the group has become most of the present world for all of you. You have had time and spent energy to get to know each other by narrative, present responses, gestures, habits, mannerisms, quirks, constant exchange, and then changes and developments.

Faced with the outgroup, the *self-definition* that was so important for people *within* the group at first, has now become *group-definition*, in the face of the outsiders. There are differences. One is that you have become wiser through the first process, the intragroup one, which you have examined in detail. Another is the size of projective screen offered by a whole other group, rather than a few other individuals. Broader brushstrokes can be applied, and representation may be much less accurate than within the group.

The Ecology Conference, not surprisingly, seems to have emerged as a Good Group, probably in part because it has massive overlap of values with yours. Too, they sound a younger group, and are more newly arrived, and self-confessedly ignorant of group dynamics. The power balance is not threatening to you.

But the point has been reinforced, that meetings between groups are delicately emotional, with great potentiality for misunderstanding and disaster. Belief in an underlying unitedness need not be at odds with recognition of the separateness of group and group, and the possibilities of fear-generated responses between them if the process of their contact is not studied with respect and imagination.

References

Berkowitz L. and Walster E. (1976) Equity theory: towards a general theory of social interaction. In L. Berkowitz (Ed.), *Advances in Experimental Social Psychology*, Vol. 9. New York: Academic Press.

Blake R.R. and Mouton J.S. (1964) *The Managerial Grid*. Houston: Gulf Publishing.

Buss A.H. and Portnoy N.W. (1967) Pain tolerance and group identification. *Journal of Personality and Social Psychology* **6**: 106–108.

Byrne D. (1971) *The Attraction Paradigm*. New York: Academic Press.

Cartwright D. and Zander. A. (1968) *Group Dynamics*, 3rd Ed. London: Tavistock.

Festinger L., Schachter S and Back K. (1950) *Social Pressures in Informal Groups*. New York: Harper.

Gleick J. (1988) *Chaos. Making a New Science*. London: Heinemann.

Knopf D. (1991) *Gestalt in Education*. Paper presented at the 5th British Gestalt Conference at Newbattle, Scotland.

Lewin K. (1948) *Resolving Social Conflicts*. New York: Harper.

McDougall W. (1921) *The Group Mind*. Cambridge University Press.

Perls F. (1947) *Ego, Hunger and Aggression*. London: Allen and Unwin.

Samuels S. (1971) Stroke strategy. 1: The basis of therapy, *Transactional Analysis Journal* **1**.

Schumacher E. (1973). *Small is Beautiful: Economics As If People Mattered*. New York: Harper and Row.

Sherif M. and Sherif C.W. (1969) *Social Psychology*. New York: Harper and Row.

Simmel G. (1950) *The Sociology of Georg Simmel*, Ed. K. Wolff, New York: The Free Press.

Turner J.C. (1986) *Rediscovering The Social Group. A Self-Categorization Theory*. Oxford: Basil Blackwell.

Wilder D.A. (1981) Perceiving persons as a group: categorization and intergroup relations. In: D.L. Hamilton (Ed.), *Cognitive Processes in Stereotyping and Intergroup Behaviour*. Hillsdale: Erbaum.

Worchel S., Axsom D., Ferris F., Samaha C. and Schweitzer S. (1978). Factors determining the effect of intergroup co-operation on intergroup attraction. *Journal of Conflict Resolution* **22**.

Chapter 14

Friday afternoon: The wider gestalt

Jan writes: This account illustrates even more graphically than the last, the early part of post-contact. The whole organism of each of you is re-organising to assimilate a plethora of new learning, and mourn, to deal with ending. Fore-contact to new gestalts is implicit in the process. The group has vanished, and its traces are carried in each member, ineradicable, however applied, interpreted or scotomised.

Post-contact will arguably be finished for Grace when she has stopped thinking about the group, and is doing some of what her presence at it has prompted her to begin. By then the digestive, selective, assimilative phase will be over, and the learning from the group will be part of her physiology rather than her awareness.

It just struck me between the eyes once more as I read this piece that, except for Sohan, the whole lot of you were brought up in cultures which lay much greater emphasis on individual than on group. Some of what you have struggled with, or come on in moments of brilliant insight during this week, are just ordinary assumptions for the majority of people in the world. China is a Far Eastern example of a group-centred consciousness. So are the myriad cultures still in touch with their tribal origins. So I remind myself of the spadework I often want to overlook in working with any collection of Westerners. Or most, anyway. Denial can be the starting point, and swooning over-identification with just one present group the worst scenario end point in a lot of the group training you and I set up.

It is worth saying again: a massive loss to most people in what is called the developed world, is neglect of the *sense of belonging*. The reality is heterogeneity, membership of a rich variety of groups. The actuality I find is very often life in single or one family accommodation. Consulting with organisations, I often come across a sense of not belonging at all, or of belonging to one room or department, which needs to defend itself against the rest of the system, rather than contribute to and be fed by that system.

Membership of cities or countries is often experienced as no more than the obligation to pay taxes and be subject to restrictive laws. This alienation is increased by mobility. Then when there is an outgroup threat, the sense of national or race membership springs out like a mad thing and leads to annihilating acts.

With this background, there is little wonder you, like many small groups in experiential training, have allowed yourselves such intensity of experience in the small temporary system you made at Hartley Manor. The experience of affiliation (Leary 1957) has probably been far more rarely sustained and enhanced in your experience before this group, than its opposite, hostility.

In her anti-racist work, Grace probably has more insight than many of you, into inadequate sense of group, and consequent pathological group behaviour. At a wide level, she works for social change already. What she is now experiencing with extreme discomfort is the inadequacy of some of her own group memberships, along with a need to let go of certain prized identities, such as what she terms *black wonder kid*. This definition of herself is as an outsider, a maverick. A paradox is that many you are outsiders in this culture, in your devotion to the topic of groups. You are loners for perhaps having the belief I do, that Cartwright and Zander, Miller and Rice, Moreno, Bion, Schutz, are scholars whose findings might with massive advantage be introduced to more of school education than an occasional liberal experiment. That is what I call the wide gestalt of where experiential group work needs to be introduced.

These are not Grace's thoughts, as she experiences in her person what are in great measure systemic faults, functions of the environment. By the time you read this, I guess most of you will know that Grace ended up taking some time out back in the Caribbean this late autumn. And she and I are doing my Greek workshops together this coming summer. I guess her gift to us was this

The wider gestalt

reminder that the heady experience possible in one-off groups is not a substitute for the monitoring and reality-testing and affiliative feeling of belonging to more enduring small support systems.

Grace's account

It's Sunday, and everyone has gone out, so I'm sitting bleak in an empty house, missing the group, and yet still feeling reluctant to put on the tape and bring back what will be a crude two-dimensional record of our last afternoon. I think of the other write-ups which are in my case still, and wonder if anyone will read them. Or whether it would be a good idea to do so. As far as I know, Birde was the only one who read them all through as they were produced.

She was the one who made a toast in orange juice at our last lunch, which we ate as a group picnic under the walnut tree, it was so stifling inside. She said, "To our expanding selves!" We drank, then made the predictable jokes about the food and getting fat.

Annie touched Birde's face and said, "I have taken in some of your passion to understand, and expanded myself with that." Birde smiled back at her. Spontaneously, we continued telling how we had used each other, in reward exchanges (Thibaut and Kelley 1959) for what Perls would call excitement and growth.

The first figure for me was the added sense of competence I had made for myself, by learning more about the analytic climate of opinion from Pierre. Perls' objections to free association (Perls, Hefferline and Goodman 1951), to Freud's topological description of the psyche, and whatnot, often obscure how much Gestalt is rooted in his analytic training. I've often joined in the chiyiking, without knowing enough what I was talking about. Now I've done some more chewing, and have more discrimination in accepting or rejecting for myself.

Annie said that for the first time in her life she knew the potential of the therapeutic group. "I know that this was not meant as a therapeutic group. But we have used it for healing and for changing. I am not sure if that is therapy, or life, or if there is a useful distinction to be made between them."

Sappho fidgeted and then said, "I could speak of very emotional things here. But more, I reflect on whether I need my personality any more. Yes, I am still so egocentric, you will think. But in future I think I know also how to be more like Annie, more like Grace. You do not need to remind us all at every moment of your identity, as I do." As each person spoke, I could see very well what they meant. But I would not have been able to forecast any of these statements.

Chuck said that the personal learning about his childhood and its effect, would probably stay most with him. He added, "Sappho gave me some out-of-class help with that, too."

Sohan said that he had learned so much each day that it was impossible for him to choose one thing. Birde said that she saw a gain in authority in him. I said that I suspected Sohan was a light still slightly under a bushel. He might have had authority all the time; but we had cast him as timid, and he had partly taken on that personality at first. He assured us earnestly that this was not so. Dear old Sohan. Well he would, wouldn't he?

I was massively aware of Orminda and Pierre, who had not spoken. The anxiety was there in me that they were just deflating, sinking away from each other as the end of the group rushed at us. It looked that way. Orminda said, "You know what I have had from this group. Of course there've been all the intellectual things. But when I arrived here I was Kay in *The Snow Queen*, and you were Gerda, who melted the piece of ice in my heart." Sohan asked to understand the story, and she added, "Kay was carried off by the Snow Queen and imprisoned in her cold palace. Little Gerda." She stopped speaking and cried for a second. She did not say that she had momentarily remembered another little girl, her dead child. I supposed she had, and I think we all did. That is the beauty of a group with continuous time together. Communication is so easy.

She went on speaking, "Gerda cared enough about him to go and find him. I think it was her kiss, or it might have been her tears, that melted the ice."

"There has been so much melting here, for me too," said Birde.

Then we waited in silence for Pierre. At last he raised his eyes to meet Orminda's, and said, "You have given me back my heart and my balls."

Startlingly, Chuck gave a loud whoop and said, "Right on! So what are you going to do about it, cobber?"

"It is not clear to me," said Pierre. "We have to move on." I don't remember how we broke up, at this point, who it was who started clearing dishes or talking about ordering taxis. But we edged away.

Our bags were all in the hall since after breakfast. I remember seeing them at this time, and aching to go. It was like the feeling I used to get at Christmas as a child, when it was evening, and the grown-ups started to quarrel. I could not bear to have the Christmas memory spoilt, and I would take a new book up to my room. And then be shouted at for not helping with the supper.

Sappho and Chuck arrived last, back at the walnut tree. Sohan then said, "I should like to ask that in this last session we hold faithfully to the Gestalt rule of speaking in the true present tense. It is a good practice for me when I am again in my art classes." He paused and added, "I am aware of a strange mental state. Early this morning I walked to the village, and I worry myself, remembering how I twice mistook people there for members of this group." Pierre quoted Patrick Casement on transference (1985), and Orminda got him to translate himself into the present, and add in his own feelings.

"I am full of the wish for us all to meet again," said Sohan, much more proactive than usual. There was a lot of argument over whether we were avoiding the end by such a plan. But we did agree on a follow-up day in London next February. This had been in Jan's original plan. We said we would invite him. I was devious here. On the phone on Thursday morning, Jan had offered this February meeting, at no charge, if we wanted it. But I never reported this. I think I was protecting you, Jan. Now the group owns the idea. It is not your imposition.

"It will not be the same," said Birde. "This group will never be the same again. It is not likely that we shall all attend such a meeting, however much we think we shall. So we must say the real goodbye this afternoon."

"Before we do that," replied Sohan, as unpredictable in his way of ending as Manfred had been, "I am wishing to tell and to hear the changes we imagine we shall make to our lives."

"What about staying in the present?" Chuck asked.

"I quote to you," said Sohan with satisfaction, taking a broken copy of *Gestalt Therapy* (Perls, Hefferline and Goodman 1961) from the cloth bag he carries: *"Memories and prospects are present imaginations. The warm play of imagination is in general not dissociative but integrative."* He read with emphasis, even relish, so that several of us smiled. Manfred's legacy of on-the-spot references had finally reached the last of the males, and an unlikely one. Then he outlined a most ambitious study plan for himself, which Annie helped him reduce to an application to the Open University for a prospectus. I thought how I would miss this monitoring, reality-testing aspect of living in this group. So I found myself saying, "I live three lives, one in my work, one with my children and relatives, and one with lovers. I have no peer group, because the lovers never seem anything to do with therapy. Can I phone some of you sometimes?"

"Please speak Gestalt," said Sohan.

"I'm imagining the comfort of phoning Annie and maybe having lunch with her, or Chuck. Even the rest of you overseas when it's cheap rate," I said obediently.

"Sohan is being monitor. The last day or so we have not had one, and we have been lax over some of the disciplines of Gestalt," said Annie. "I shall go on working at how to make the tasks and roles in groups clear. In practice, it does not seem enough to say simply that we are all responsible for ourselves."

"Yet," said Chuck, "this group has been anarchic by chance, and it sure looks as good a blueprint as I could come up with in how to educate people into Anarchy with a big A. The whole damn thing is about awareness. I know and you know what we're doing to ourselves. And what our effect is on each other. Sure, we're not evolved enough yet to be good Anarchists for long. But I'm damned if I want to go in for role clarity as if it was preferable to the anarchic thing. Specialised roles work. But they diminish flexibility in everyone. OK, translating to Gestalt, I am dreaming of a ward one day where I spell out the old Awareness and Responsibility code to the patients, then I and the staff mostly get on with what *we* want to do there, which for me probably means, commenting on the contact processes between people. After all, pretty well all psychological distress is to do with what you Gestalties call the contact processes."

I remembered, aloud, the resistance there had been to Gestalt at the beginning of the week. Now there was a process going on that vaguely reminded me of Balinese people bringing offerings. Were we bargaining, offering propitiations to some Nemesis of

The wider gestalt

Gestalt, who might otherwise strike us down when we went back to the savage world?

The next bit I recall is Pierre saying, "There is a contradiction in Gestalt. Perls speaks of growth in the human personality, in the title of his book (Perls 1951). But he also states in it that *In ideal circumstances the self does not have much personality. It is the sage of Tao that is 'like water' assuming the form of the receptacle* (p. 427). Before you interrupt me, Grace, I wish to say that I consider you nearer this personality-free self of Perls' description, than any other person here." He was giving a compliment in his tortuous way, and one I am not clear whether I merit or not. But he too was bringing his little offering, albeit with a sour lemon slice in it, to the altar of Gestalt.

"I cannot bear this," said Sappho. "I cannot bear to go on that plane and to suffocate to death in the pollution of Athens, and to leave Chuck."

"Please use Gestalt language," said Sohan, and she started again. "I feel something like a tearing in my heart. My legs and shoulders are weak. I push myself to make bad images of Athens, and only idealised images of this group." She smiled wryly, and said "Aha."

"Just this requirement, to describe the inner process accurately, is a therapeutic miracle," said Birde, adding to Sohan, "There. Now you are an advanced Gestalt practitioner."

"No," said Sohan, "for that I need also to disclose my process as I speak."

There was a pause, and Chuck said, "What are we doing? I feel the involvement. But I can't describe the process."

"To understand process, first notice the context, the environment," said Orminda. "We are dealing with the departure. Whatever we talk about or do, the context is that. And the way we are doing it seems a bit as Grace suggested, a homage to Gestalt. We have a reprise of this theme and that. I think we are offering each other, and ourselves, proofs that we have learned. They are the proofs that we have valued each other, and that we have been Chuck's cannibals, who magically eat each other and go away the more expanded. So this is the end of the beginning."

Before I knew, or almost before I knew what I was doing, I said, "Pierre, you and Orminda need to stay in touch."

"And how is this interesting statement part of Gestalt?" he

replied quickly, knee-jerked into his old contemptuous defensive style.

"It's called awareness-raising," I said grandly, and would say no more. Nobody supported me. I could not tell whether this was from a wise judgement that he would become yet more defensive; or because they did not share my view. Perhaps I have projected all my own interest in Pierre on to Orminda, and want her to have him for me. In this strange churning of all my ideas since I came home, I have already lost certainty about that.

Chuck changed the subject abruptly, by asking Sohan to join him in a research project. They would each set up two groups, structured in different ways they would describe in detail before beginning. But in essence, one would be with one of them there as leader. The other would be a peer group of patients only, given a space and time and a written description of the task, as this group had had. Sohan looked so pleased. Then Birde said:

"Now we move to the future again, to these beginnings Orminda mentioned. One little dream I have is that you all come to Gotland, a beautiful island off Sweden, and we live there together and write a book of our understandings. Well, perhaps one day when we are old!"

I said, "Dreaming is free," and she went on, more confidently, "I have thought often of Manfred and Pierre's scorn that we have no clear developmental theory in Gestalt. I have this idea to set up a Gestalt baby observation programme for my students for all this coming year. I will write all of how I do it. A phenomenological–existential dialogue approach, with careful recording. That will be my baby." We all talked eagerly of this, offering ideas and counter-ideas.

"There's an almost frightened excitement in my insides," said Annie, "as I see us picking up the Gestalt baton and running with it. If Chuck goes back to Australia next year, that means that these influences we are turning into, will run all over the globe. Scandinavia, Greece. I wish Manfred was still here. By the way, I have a spare bedroom and plenty of space for anyone who wants to stay in London."

"What an interesting juxtaposition of subjects," said Pierre, and she blushed.

"What I thought I was setting out to say," she went on, "was that I am still a toddler in Gestalt. So I shall do nothing more

The wider gestalt

innovative than take a course in it when I am back in London. But I am a different toddler, a child of this group. This is my infancy of a different life, parented by you, and parented by who I was before." Many of us nodded. I recognised that this applied to me. But so often the other people have been figural for me here, that I have been self-neglectful, and forgotten to make an ambition on my own account. That is not true presence, to be so aware of what is outside as to ignore what is inside. No wonder it is so dreary to sit here now. I will phone Annie in a minute. We might go for an Indian meal or something.

There's a line in an Adrian Mitchell poem, *Scrub my skin with women*. It's about anaesthetising yourself with sensation. Maybe I must live this one out without a fuck, or a chat over a restaurant table. I need a major realignment to change from being the black wonder kid to the wise woman.

Not getting Pierre was probably the healthiest thing that happened to me at Hartley Manor. Poor Birde, with whom I avoided identifying. I think she may be going through the same lonely process as me. But she has her little plan already, for a Gestalt experiment, a new departure. I just have the vile writhings of discomfort with what is, the golden memory of what was last week, and the temptation to choose the old path of depression, rather than face change. All my sexiness gone, Jan. All my jaunty flirting is in some bin of dismalness.

Jan's comment

I ask myself if Grace was perhaps going through the uncomfortable but healthy process described by Perls, Hefferine and Goodman (1951, on p. 413):

> The weak figures lose interest and become confused, the self loses its "security" and suffers. Yet this suffering is not a weakening of the self, but a painful transitional excitement of creativity.

Like many people after a residential group, she is suddenly back in the very environment which supported or produced some of the attitudes and behaviours she wants to change. It is a bit like retiring to a fish and chip shop to begin a fat-free diet, or to a Trappist monastery to try out your dialogic skills. This dislocation tests the post-contact, assimilative abilities, rather than enhances them. So there is the strongest case for designing follow-up to residential groups which have therapy, change or growth in their agendas.

You have made yourselves a telephone network, as well as various pairings, and the formal meeting in six or seven months, as a social method for dealing with the beginning of post-contact. Rather than see these as an avoidance of the end, as Pierre from his training might well have done, a more Gestalt perception might be that these devices are also a way of preserving the whole of the group. People do end and die. Groups such as families and racial groups may, but are not doomed to do the same. This is to me an important possibility to remember when I see what might in other theories be called resistance to the ending of a group.

The last meeting of the group contained many statements about present learning and change. Yet the feel, from the account, is of excited moving forward, the making of new appetites for new experiences. One way to describe some of this is in terms of *unfinished gestalts*.

The nearest example is Grace, who suspects that she suppressed her own desire for Pierre. She made sense of it as a symptom of a general lack of intellectual as well as carnal companionship in her life. Nevertheless, she has neither paired fully with Pierre, found another partner, nor moved to a different view of the field. She is left questing for a new creative adjustment.

From an outsider's view, it looks likely that you have all carried away a litter of unfinished gestalts, likely to result in creative turmoil for a time. One, only glimpsed in the last part of the week, was to do with the abrupt changes of perception of the field, once other groups have entered it. Me-and-the-rest-of-the-group was the whole field very often, in the early phases. The group-in-Hartley-Manor was another important field. Only with the inter-group meetings did people begin to notice clearly that the dynamic whole of the group had its own boundary. Within this, you construed yourselves as one-of-this-group in relation to one-of-that-group. Idiosyncracy was less salient than group membership. The performance or honour or status of The Group took precedence over that of the individual.

In this reduction of individuality, and in the shifting context of task and meeting, to some extent a caricature of elements of

The wider gestalt

personality of the members, emerged. In the encounter with the Counselling Group, your competitive aggression was strongly exaggerated. In the tabula rasa encounter with the Ecology Group, your considerable leadership and teaching skills were in evidence. Competitive motives were probably there, but had found a creative and functional expression, which made reward for both groups. As we have now established, you reckon that you did not at the time see yourselves as a competitive lot. Had I been there, I guess you would have done. Unless strong characteristics are up in awareness, they can seem to leap at you in a pretty uncomfortable way.

I think you kind of knew your group character, or you would not perhaps have been so careful in your plans to meet the other groups, second time round. But sort of knowing is only second best to being well aware. And I, and Gestalt, are about raising awareness. Maybe there is more to do even than that. I would like to say some more about this in my endpiece to what looks like turning into a book.

Contact skills between groups are one of the most urgently needed skills, if human survival is of interest. There are probably re-educative stages needed. The intrapersonal needs to be tended sufficiently before contact with others can be flexible and socially rewarding. In the same way, the intra-group requires proper attention before there is any possibility of enough insight for a healthy group sense. Only then is inter-group contact likely to be other than a caricature of the fears of group members. The neurologist Kurt Goldstein's statement (1939), that *behaviour is always organised, and always implicates the whole organism*, is of as lively interest at group at personal level. The group, like a person, will behave in the light of its deficiency needs, until these have been attended to enough to allow the growth needs into awareness (Goldstein 1939; Maslow 1954).

At the time of writing, the splintering of the USSR, of the ethnic sub-groups of Iraq, of Yugoslavia, Spain, Afghanistan. Somalia, testify to a rising global awareness of group identity, characterised at the moment by narrow gestalting, fragmentation, and by a brutality of inter-group contact which is in grotesque contrast to the friendship and respect which was there between member and member of many of the groups before.

This is the world to which you returned. It is no wonder that Birde dreamed of the cocoon of goodness (Anzieu 1975), of making an international community where her new friends could pursue some ideal existence, away from the outgroup.

There is not a tidy sinking down of the group as a figure of interest, in a copybook show of post-contact. The week will be the talisman of some of you for years to come. The experiences you had within it may come to fruition as insights in a month or six months or a year, or longer.

At a simple level, one important and not often mentioned function of a group has been well demonstrated. It is, to stimulate, to energise its members. And the stimulation can be so upsetting, that I have made my mind up to ask anyone joining a short course of mine, what support groups exist for them in the rest of their life. If they have none, I will not accept them. Grace has shown me enough to make me secure of saying that. She is a very talented woman with maybe more charisma than is good for her. Of course you all made her queen of the group at the start of it. And of course she put the crown aside with a smile, the way she always does: she knows she will be offered it again. But this time, she was toppled from being most-desirable-female. And what she did was to give up being most-dominant-female too. If her group position or role faltered in one respect, out went the lot, as far as I can puzzle. That is something none of you noticed enough at the time to make useful sense of. It is a wound that needs reparative treatment, probably in a home-group where the people know the bewildered returning member. And Grace, the person as well known as any among you for her group work, has no support group of her own. The cobbler's child is always the worst shod.

As in most groups of this intensity and brevity, one possibility is that the challenge to change that Grace, or any other member has experienced, is so great and so full of discomfort, that it will be seen as unattainable, and jettisoned completely, baby and bathwater. Pierre, Orminda, Grace, Annie, Birde, and to a lesser extent Sappho and Sohan, have seen the need for major shifts in the whole way they live. But the old ways will beckon and nudge at them. Will a few letters or telephone calls be support enough to keep their courage for change? The meeting in February will give some evidence. If it is made to happen.

References

Anzieu D. (1975) *The Group and the Unconscious.* Trans. B. Kilborne. London: Routledge and Kegan Paul, 1984.
Bion W. (1961) *Experiences in Groups.* London: Tavistock.
Cartwright D. and Zander A., (1968) *Group Dynamics*, 3rd Ed. New York: Harper and Row.
Casement P. (1985) *On Learning from the Patient.* London: Tavistock.
Goldstein K. (1939) *The Organism.* Boston: American Book Co.
Leary T. (1957) *The Interpersonal Diagnosis of Personality.* New York: Ronald.
Maslow A. (1954) *Motivation and Personality.* New York: Harper.
Miller E. (Ed.) (1976) *Task and Organization.* London: John Wiley.
Mitchell A. (1991) To whom it may concern. In: *Adrian Mitchell's Greatest Hits.* Newcastle upon Tyne: Bloodaxe Books.
Perls F., Hefferline R. F. and Goodman P. (1951) *Gestalt Therapy. Excitement and Growth in the Human Personality.* New York: Dell.
Schutz W. (1958) *The Interpersonal Underworld.* Palo Alto: Science and Behaviour Books, 1966.
Thibaut J. W. and Kelley H. H. (1959) *The Social Psychology of Groups.* New York: John Wiley.

Chapter 15

The follow-up: Assimilation, new awareness, and beginnings

Jan writes: So it happened! I got to meet you! I feel such an elation, remembering our day at Annie's London home last week. Pictures stay in my mind as I write. One is of Pierre's son, Jean-Jacques of the skinny legs and big boots, leaving his drawing and coming to sit in the group, leaning against Orminda. Another is of the empty chair set for Sappho. Then there was the occupied chair that was Manfred's, to the great pleasure and surprise of more than just me. And so for the first time I am facing what each of you has already had to decide when you were scribe, of whether to start with the story of what everyone said and did, or jump straight at the ideas behind or around what was going on.

I've just come on notes I made way back last spring, of some structures meant to help us frame what was happening in the group. First of these had to be Lewin's field theory, already so closely associated with Gestalt. Then I remembered Herschel's original Scientific Model:

- *First, make observations, ask questions and seek explanations.* (This you did.)
- *Second, construct an explanatory model.* (You did this, tentatively and piecemeal.)
- *Third, examine the adequacy of the model by applying it to new data, and wherever possible, to data derived from experiment.* (In the group you were at too early a stage to do that. But the

Assimilation, new awareness, and beginnings   203

writing of Chuck, Sohan and Birde since, shows that has been happening too, in very creative and co-operative experiments with patients and students.)

Later than that, just half a century ago, Cartwright and Zander (1953) asked four questions they saw as central to proceeding with research and training in group dynamics:

1. *What is the proper relationship between data-collecting and theory building?*
2. *What are the proper objects of study and techniques of observation?*
3. *What are the basic variables that determine what happens in groups?*
4. *How can the many factors affecting group life be combined into a comprehensive conceptual system?*

How pleasant, and how impossible, to find four neat answers. But in an emergent, inchoate way I can feel the pattern and rhythm of a Gestalt answer, specially to the last question. That is the excitement to me of seeing you work away at relating the personal, particular, often unique and profound personal experiences of your group, to the great flux of forming and re-forming groups throughout the life of every human.

Eleanor O'Leary's chapter on "Methods, issues and new directions in gestalt therapy" (O'Leary 1992) gives informed suggestions for systemised research, which will go beyond the studies of Foulds and Hannigan (1977), Côté (1982) and Swain (1989).

So I have started this piece with ideas, before I noticed what I was doing. Slow down, Padrewski.

I heard from Annie as soon as I was back in the States last autumn, inviting me to the follow-up. I accepted, a little uncomfortably, wondering if this was to be a Day of Judgement on me. Then Grace sent me the write-ups of the sessions, and I felt that I was coming to know you all in a most intimate way, as I added bits of commentary, and felt shifts in my own understanding and feelings. I stopped fearing you. Instead, I think I entered into creative competition with you, and began to hone my offering to the group, reminiscent of the offerings some of you had made or envisaged at the last meeting at Hartley. Ideas that have lain round my mind like half-written pieces of music have been hauled out and laboured over. Yeah, if competition is the name of the game, I'm in there.

Or maybe it's emulation I'm talking about, a showing I can do well too. These ideas are not there to bat yours down. They are made in part from yours, and from your writings about the week. Co-creation. *In the individual's mental life someone else is invariably involved, as a model, as an object, as a helper, as an opponent; and so from the very first individual psychology ... is at the same time social psychology as well* (Freud 1921). That's Freudian for what Lewin and Perls and the rest of the Gestaltists express as the indivisibility of figure and field.

The contact helix

The business of each is to preserve and enhance its wholeness. I write that in italics, since it was one of the hypotheses we all agreed on at our day together. Preserving wholeness comes first, whether of individual, sub-group, or whatever configuration is foreground. Enhancing, growing, can happen where conditions are perceived as favourable for that to happen. This way of giving meaning to what have usually been called resistances to contact just feels right to me. Curiously, these reflections give a different emphasis for me to that embarrassing Gestalt prayer: I do my thing and you do your thing, and if we meet, that's wonderful. I can hear that now with the sub-text of all the peril and complication of each person's preserving their own wholeness. Then it seems really wonderful that any of us survive the battering of the world, to meet and light up and enrich each other, the way you people so signally did last summer and since.

We have met, deeply. What I write here is a function of you, the group, and me. And one of the creative adjustments I am making in response to what I have learned from you, is a new version of that old Cycle of Experience that has been a useful teaching aid these many years. Ed and Sonia Nevis's depictions of a wave form of interactive cycle were in my mind, part of the field too, sparked by Grace's commentary in Session Ten.

I saw two lines, one for I, one for Thou. The lines are like wave energy, which is also particles, matter. Seen as a particle, I and Thou could be shown as circles, formed by a contact boundary

Assimilation, new awareness, and beginnings

that will be osmotically permeable at times, and solid, for purposes of rejection and self-preservation, at other times. The particle could even be seen as a cross-section of the line.

The wave particles that are two organisms may make a spiral, a double helix, overlapping in contact, then parting in withdrawal. As I visualise this diagram, it can be varied to give a subjective representation of any particular contact, between two people, or two groups. The different depictions by each party might be a fast diagnosis of a failure of communication. I include a diagram, on page 206, to show more of what I mean.

Apart or a part

So what else have you confessed to making yourselves aware of, through this profound episode last summer and onwards?

You learned more about that continuing chicken and egg enigma of group and individual. Are you as an individual no more than a nodal point, a role or Lewinian dynamic in many consecutive presents, expressing what in that configuration needs to be expressed? Are you a carrier of the emotions and responses of the group, with only illusory free will? You have told me how you came to understand more profoundly than before, the extent to which your feelings, and feelings for each other, were a product of the various and complex environments you separately perceived and responded to. Yet no, you seem not to have decided that you were puppets of fate. But you have an enhanced respect for the power of the group in determining your awareness.

I have a fine letter from Manfred in which he traces again the ancient group consciousness he transferred on to the Hartley experience. The pattern of what I could call Orminda's Joan of Arc syndrome, her putting herself forward to do a service for the group at great personal expense, is another example of this. You could all probably cite your own instances. You found that you did not just transfer old scenes to the new one. You cast a role for yourself and at least some of the others, and worked hard to get everyone to act the familiar scenes.

DIAGNOSTIC PATTERN OF CONTACT
[To be drawn by both parties to an interaction]

EXAMPLE: Chuck and Sappho's week together, configured as one interaction (Sappho's version))

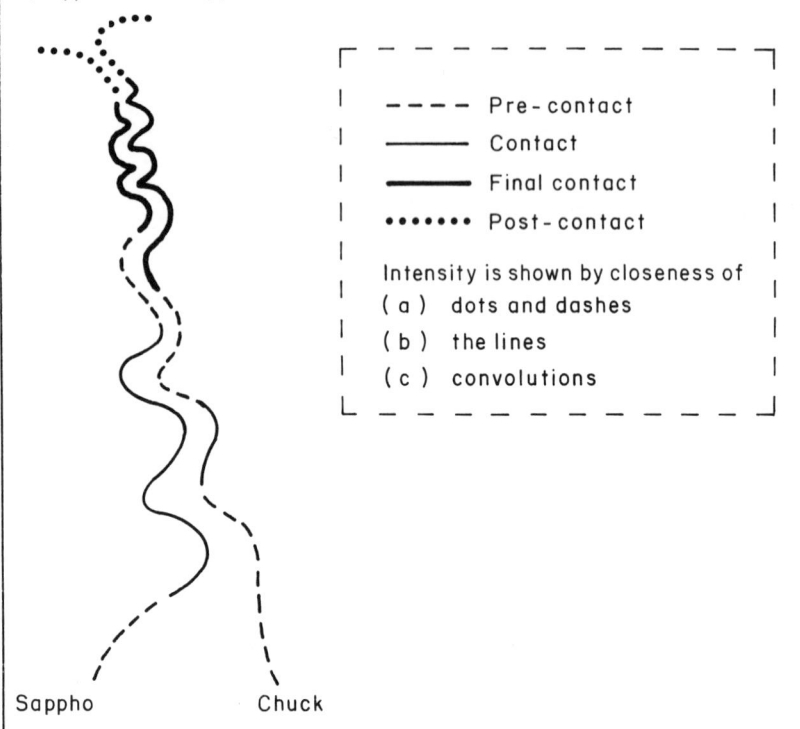

```
- - - -   Pre-contact
———       Contact
━━━       Final contact
••••••    Post-contact
```

Intensity is shown by closeness of
(a) dots and dashes
(b) the lines
(c) convolutions

Sappho   Chuck

The line in the diagram can be expressed as a particle or cross-section:

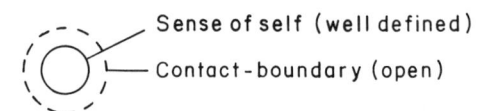

— Sense of self (well defined)
— Contact-boundary (open)

From moment to moment, or person to person, the gap between self and contact-boundary, and the nature of the two, will be perceived in many different combinations; e.g.:

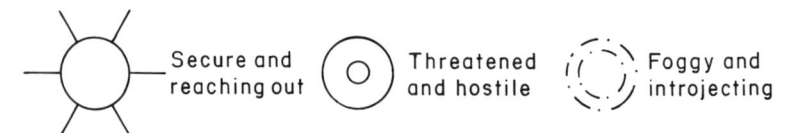

Secure and reaching out   Threatened and hostile   Foggy and introjecting

Transference and projective identification

I have used the word transference again. Do you remember that moment when Sohan said he had seen several of you in the village, though you were at Hartley all the time? We could say, in Gestalt language, he projected his perception of you on to some other people. I would rather acknowledge an excellent concept from psychoanalysis, and say he transferred. To me, we all seem to do it all day long.

A newly formed group is an inter-group event to me. The members, like actors in full costume, studied in the lines from one of their repertoire of plays, search for a Hamlet to their Ophelia, a gangster to their policeman, and come instead, perhaps, on Figaros or Scarlett O'Haras. Even more interestingly, a determined playing of any of these roles may actually get the other actors joining in, in ways that may be unfamiliar, gratifying or highly alarming to them. I would like to let in to Gestalt the term *transference*, using it to sum up this taking of any historic position, not just one of infant to parent, and the attempt to elicit complementary dynamics or roles from others.

Projective identification is used differently by various writers. I like the sense of it that makes a neat extension of the gestalt *projection*: I project; if you identify heavily with what I am projecting at you, that is a projective identification. Then we surely start to play a scene that I have rehearsed before, which might not be an experience of any excitement and growth for either of us, and might leave you feeling used. You have been.

Determinism

One question you were dealing with time and again during your week, as you compared theories, remembered apposite comments by many writers, was whether any systems are archetypal. In other words, you faced yourselves with the possibility that, say, a group of a certain size with a certain kind of task will almost inevitably go through certain predictable processes.

Pierre, one of the more determinist members, who at times seemed sure of the meaning of some group behaviour more or less before it happened, has written a lot to me of his new understanding of the effect of environment, present context and structure, on perception and behaviour. Conversely, Birde has been discovering in her winter workshops, the discernible evolutionary phases that recapitulate from one small group to another, time and again, though by no means inevitably.

These phases could be from slime to mammal, from womb to three months, from birth to adulthood, from childhood to death, from infancy to leaving home. I hope you are noticing all the contradictory stages that any one group can be accused of living through.

From what you said last week, it sounds like most of you are settling for there being a shape or pattern that each group seems to make between its start and its end, *if it has one*. Gestalt is concerned with noticing what model, if any discernible one, is being used by a particular group at a particular time. This seems to me a more useful position than assuming that all small groups will do the Kleinian thing or the Freudian or Sternian thing or whatever. Maybe there are archetypes. Maybe there are a lot of them, like there were a lot of gods and goddesses tumbling around on Olympus, getting up to a stack of behaviours we could copy. The work I give myself is to know as many of these myths or group theories as I can. Then I may usefully notice which, if any, seem operant in a present group. After all, humans need models to understand things by.

In commenting on your sessions, I got fond of the Stern analogy, of fancying the group to make a collective version of *emergent*, *core*, *intersubjective* and *narrative self*. Birde favours the buzz-words *Dependence*, *Counter-Dependence*, *Independence* and *Interdependence* to describe the possible evolution of a group (Houston 1984). I hope she keeps the idea as a map rather than an inevitable prediction. To my mind, by the way, it certainly looks as if your, or now our, group has in that schema got to interdependence. I feel myself a sibling, not even *primus inter pares*, when I see how you have already picked up and run with the learning you got last summer. Chuck and Sohan have already extended their hospital experiments, and look all set to publish something together at the end of the year. I'm excited about that.

By and large, theories of group behaviour which stress chronological stages are more determinist than those that speak, as Schutz, Bion and others have, of various positions or group tasks.

Assimilation, new awareness, and beginnings

Perls offers us a magnificent model of how to see into the depths of now, the instant, and read in this microcosm all that is there. *The present moment holds the seeds of the future, and is as well the culmination of the whole of the past.* The originality of every person is as great a truth as that we often do the same things in the same kinds of scene. *There is far less behaviour possible than motivation.*

Group contact boundary

An awareness many of you have been digesting, or maybe still savouring before swallowing, is of the group contact boundary. Even an idiosyncratic rivalrous lot like you could be sprung into some notion of having a group identity, a contact boundary which contained the lot of you. Manfred helped at experiential level with that. At theory level, his open systems ideas, of the organic need for small primary groups in all human systems, is totally in line with mine.

The boundary is subtly delineated between, and by, what is coming from outside, and the state of receptivity of what is inside. So, though the idea of a boundary is perfectly understandable to all of you, the exact delineation of it is more elusive. In the same way, the boundary of a group becomes clear to its members when the environment creates the necessary contrast for that clarity. But there is no chalk line or bag of skin or whatever round any group. A sceptic might say that we are talking here of no more than a myth. Well, I am not too worried if anyone does call the group contact boundary a myth. It is as powerful a myth as any I can recall. What is more, it is one of those central concepts in Gestalt, that is probably the most illuminating to our understanding of group behaviour. For example, you seemed to know, even before anyone quoted you the experiments and theory, that you would get the other group to reinforce its boundary to fortress status if you arrived in a solid phalanx. Yet sending one representative roused your paranoia and your protectiveness of your envoy. If it was difficult to manage that boundary work comfortably at a summer residential, then I see the chasm of judgement that needs to be filled, if we are to manage international, inter-racial, inter-cultural contact boundaries to better effect than we often do now.

In many scenes my perception is of being just me walking down a street or shaking someone's hand. From the reactions of others, I am bounced back to acknowledging that for them I am an envoy of some group or other, on to which they may be projecting a stack of stuff. The task may then be to convince them that I belong to an acceptable sub-set of the hated group, or to some other group altogether. Or to start changing their view of my group. Now my memory goes to how much we talked in London of the two major kinds of groups, ephemeral ones like yours, and groups like families, and all the institutions which are likely to have a much longer life than that of any member, and so for the individual are endless.

Theories as group banners

Grace's going into psychoanalysis seems to have upset Birde, who sees it as a betrayal of Gestalt. She's talking banners. A banner is useful to rally to when you risk getting lost. I think it's less use when it comes to mean if-you're-not-in-our-team-you're-a-cissy. To me, the modern, interactive analysis Grace is engaged in sounds a proper re-marriage between the analytic and Gestalt traditions. Freud's hypotheses of drives and instincts within the individual are partly verified by laboratory research. At the same time, field theory, and the primacy of intersubjective experience, is being substantiated in similar research. Grace says her analyst is in part an unaware or instinctive Gestaltist. You found that you were in part unaware Freudians and Foulkesians and systems analysts and Jungians and the Lord knows what all else. I like that, if it makes you better theorists and practitioners.

Let me just put it on the record that the brand-name is not the essence for me. I have that group-boundary consciousness that makes me splutter that this or that is pure Gestalt (which is shorthand or euphemism for *mine*) when it re-emerges within a different system. But that at worst is the stuff of flag-waving, power games and petty victories. The learning that stays with me from your inter-group experiences is to focus wider, to the broad field of all human, which is to say, all group behaviour. I can agree for example with David Levinson (1978) that no part of a system can be considered outside its context or its relatedness to other parts of the system.

Assimilation, new awareness, and beginnings

So many people from so many disciplines are in a position to contribute to one overarching understanding. And I notice weak feelings as I write, that I sure do hope that other schools will think this way too, and not claim factional victory for any breakthrough. I am not too evolved, even if hopeful of what can be. Maybe I am a readout of where we have all evolved to. We begin to have an intellectual grasp of more; and our emotionality still plays the underdog, the way you showed so clearly in reporting your premeeting near the end of the week, with the Counselling Group. You had planned how to be the perfect group; then in you went and started boasting.

Praegnanz and emergency responses

You had been fumbling towards a technology of improving intergroup contact. The scientific hypothesis might be that hostility between certain kinds of groups exists, is undeniably there, even if it can be eclipsed or suppressed temporarily.

Before you laugh me down as idealistic, I want to comment on the different competitive feelings I can experience, and I guess at being in general experience. They may be fundamental to group behaviour. They are described in different terms in Chapter 9 of Volume 2 of *Gestalt Therapy* (Perls, Hefferline and Goodman 1951). One is the spur to my writing all this, and is somehow fearless. I am keyed up, stimulated by the rest of you, and wanting both to show myself worthy of being in what is now a reference group for me, and to offer you some gift. The fearlessness is to do with supposing that if you see differently from me, or if I have my facts or ideas screwed up, your response will be to fight me, yes. Wrestling makes for good energy. But we'll be hand to hand, showing our positions, and ready to yield to a stronger one. This is different from a shootout or a psychological air strike, which annihilates.

We are back with the only two major intersubjective motivators I can ever see: love and fear. To you, My Group, I feel what I hope is a contained and discriminating love, beyond *koinonia*, De Mare's impersonal fellowship, and well short of possessiveness. The word love is so hot that a more cunning person might translate it to some partial behavioural description, like A Mode of Open

Receptivity and Approach. I notice that this makes the acronym AMORA. Neat, huh?

The Counselling Group stayed steady, in AMORA, when you retreated to fear and consequent hostility. You joined them. As Orminda looks at her country, and the inter-group fear and rage that have become culturally ingrained; as Grace reflects on the way her and other ethnic groups are treated by majority races or nations, I hope they will accept that I am being diagnostic, not prescriptive.

My tentative hypothesis is that fear leads to a simplifying of gestalt formation. This is another way of saying, a tuning out of much of the field. For example, you as a leaderless, an orphan group, got the emotional wobbles *vis-à-vis* the well-parented counsellors. There was an out-of-awareness emergency. So the emotional need for definition or recognition momentarily became greater than the overt task. In the same way, at intra-group level, you needed to define yourselves and be recognised as individuals, before you let group membership be figural.

Fear seems to create a hierarchy of gestalts of group membership itself, from being nothing, without a sense of self, as happens in crowds very often, via defining self in spite of the group, to belonging to a small group, to belonging to many groups, and being a citizen.

Belonging

I have packed so much thinking, so much of what we have written to each other about, into those few lines. I had better expand a little on some of them. Belonging to many groups is a fact of life, as we have commented. When that word is given emotional force, it illuminates personal response to this inevitability of being, say, family member, work-group member, American, Californian, and on and on.

Belonging can be experienced at the pole of fear or of AMORA. In civil war, people commonly report that factions or ethnic groups who were previously friends, become enemies. Fear of the outgroup creates a fearful and hostile clinging to the apparent safety of belonging to some designated ingroup. Another fear response to belonging is to resist it, from scare of being overwhelmed or dam-

Assimilation, new awareness, and beginnings

aged in some way. Belonging to a crowd or mob is a transitory state, complex as well as simplistic. Gross projections on to the designated enemy lead to id-level responses generating, and generated by, fear. Groups seem then like walnuts, hard and closed, and capable as a result of being smashed to fragments. These fragments can be like the Anglo-Saxon Wanderer, condemned to solitude by the loss of his lord, his kin, his feudal hall: *There is now no living man to whom I dare tell what is in my heart* (The Wanderer, in *The Exeter Book*). That sounds like a lot of people now. Except that the modern ones may not even know they have lost their belonging.

At the pole of AMORA, there is openness to growing, to giving and receiving, to enjoying rather than denying belonging. This state survives best where there is some peace, or robust confirmation of the individual or group by some of the field. In these conditions, the wide gestalt is possible. One of the many problems about sovereign groups such as governments or boards of directors or even parents, is that they may function from AMORA, while their respondent outgroups are clumping together, still fear-motivated. Unless the inter-group communication and feeling suits both, the fear-motivated groups will be the victorious underdogs.

Id and ego process

We could say that much of the work of your week together was to do with the good old Gestalt task of raising awareness. You got a grasp of the need to hold on to a definition of yourself, a shaping of your contact boundaries when you first met the others, and a need to get recognition from them. You grew aware of the emerging topics in the group, and gave yourselves the data to test whether, say, the men versus women sub-grouping is a pattern that emerges often in small groups, or was just there in yours. You got a lively awareness of the sense of group that could be sparked up, the moment another group lurched into your territory, physical or emotional. You felt the poignancy of sexual attraction, and have had leisure to work out how much of that was positional, brought about by the scene you were living, and how much was to do with longer-lasting aspects of your individual characters.

Let's be particular. Sappho's absence last week was a clear

comment, it turned out, on her loss of interest in Chuck, once she was back home. He too has got engaged to another Australian doctor this winter. He and Sappho admit they had hung their sexual and companionship needs on each other, in a Law of Praegnanz simplification that did not stand up, once the field had shifted.

It still feels a little delicate to talk of Orminda and Pierre, when his wife has so lately died. But his out-of-character boundary violation, in bringing that nice kid to the group, is not something that can be out of awareness for any of you antenna-twitching group diagnosticians.

Much brilliantly successful work is done in the name of Gestalt, addressing only ego-processes, which I could re-render here as those processes which can be readily available to awareness.

At Hartley, just so much of what you talked about could also be described as id-level, out of awareness possibilities. I reckon you partly did a regular Gestalt job, of exploring each particular behaviour or feeling, to find out more. And too, you sat and speculated about possible underlying meanings, which might give you more clues about what you were up to. Thank the Lord, you recognised speculations for what they were, and did not make them into credos or group banners to crouch under defensively and exclusively.

There is more of us below the waterline of awareness than above it, probably at iceberg proportion. I remember a line one of my students wrote: *My depths are of the same substance as my shallows*. In other words, I doubt there is anything very spooky in these id-processes, or at least, any more spooky than in the ego-processes.

The valuable and amazing capacity we have for translating from one mode to another, and transferring from one scene to another, just must mean that we variously try out whether an organisation will work like a body, or work-group like a school class, a political meeting like a Neanderthal hunting expedition, and so on.

Dreams are a route from id to ego level that Gestalt addresses. In the culture you made at Hartley, you did not explore dreams as often as you set yourselves to do. And you only looked at them for individual meaning. You dreamed within the group, though. There were social meanings and communications in your dreams that remained out of awareness.

Social dreaming, and other aspects of id-level process, need to

Assimilation, new awareness, and beginnings 215

be in the awareness of anyone who wants to develop groups to be scenes of excitement and growth. Perls spoke often of the schizophrenic levels in all of us. Losing fear of that in yourself and others, when you operate in groups, needs specialist training. To my eye, other schools have good things to offer to Gestalt in this field.

Heterogeneity

Sohan and Chuck have made a Where I Belong diagram for their patients. It shows a clear correlation between admitting belonging to many groups, and gaining self-esteem and intersubjective fluency.

Grace went back to the Caribbean to reaffirm her group of origin, that she realised she denies emotionally when in Britain. It was not enough for her to belong over in her adopted country. Width and depth are let back into identity, into the view of the world, when we let awareness move easily between our many belongings, it seems. For my money, Chuck and Sohan have lit on one of the *proper objects of study and techniques of observation* here (Cartwright and Zander 1953).

Thank you to all nine of you, if you have read this far. My excitement now, and all my thoughts, are part of a shared creativity. You are the foreground of that, on a field as vast as that vision of Annie's she told you at Hartley.

I hope I am more than just another topdog, raising his leg against the Great Lamp Post of psychological theory. John Ponting of the Gestalt Institute of Scandinavia might call me an underdog disguised as a topdog. Yes, I do want to make a mark: an invitational one. I want to go beyond a one-or-other theory of human behaviour and motivation, to that exciting region where more knowledge flickers like a newly-lighted candle in a cave, hinting by the shapes and shadows it casts at how much more there is to discover. What you are doing at best is study to illuminate the process of those discoveries, without pre-empting their content. There is the paradoxical good science of Gestalt, neither to overdetermine the problem, nor the outcome.

References

Bales R. (1950) *Interaction Process Analysis*. New York: Addison-Wesley.
Brown L. (1978) Towards a theory of power and intergroup relations. In: C. Cooper and C. Alderfer (Eds), *Advances in Experiential Social Processes*, Vol. 1. Chichester: John Wiley.
Cartwright D. and Zander A. (1953) *Group Dynamics*. London: Tavistock.
Côté N. (1982) Effects of an intensive gestalt session on the level of self-actualization and the personality structure. *Gestalt Theory* **4**: 89–106.
Erickson. E. (1951) *Childhood and Reality*. London: Imago.
Exeter Book (9th C.). Author's trans.
Foulds M. and Hannigan P. (1977) Gestalt workshop and measured changes in self-actualization; replication and refinement study. *Journal of College Student Personnel* **18**: 220–225.
Freud S. (1921) *Group Psychology and the Analysis of the Ego*. Harmondsworth: Penguin, 1991.
Houston G. (1984) *The Red Book of Groups*. London: Rochester Foundation.
Levinson D. (1978) *Seasons of a Man's Life*. New York: Knopf.
Lewin K. (1951) *Field Theory in Social Science*. New York: Harper and Row.
March J. and Simon H. (1958) *Organizations*. London: John Wiley.
O'Leary E. (1992) *Gestalt Therapy. Theory, Practice and Research*. London: Chapman and Hall.
Perls F., Hefferline R. and Goodman P. (1951) *Gestalt Therapy. Excitement and Growth in the Human Personality*. New York: Julian Press.
Stern D. (1985) *The Interpersonal World of the Infant*. New York: Basic Books.
Swain R. (1989) Effects of a seven-hour gestalt group on student self-esteem and class cohesiveness. *Journal of Higher Education Studies* **4**: 23–6.
Turquet P. (1974) Leadership, the individual and the group. In: J. Hartman and R. Mann (Eds), *Analysis of Groups*. San Francisco: Josseybass.
Zinker J. (1977) *Creative Process in Gestalt Therapy*. New York: Brunner-Mazel.

Index

Abstinence, 47, 53
Acculturation, 156
Acting out, 92
Adler, 18
Adolescence, 138
Affect, 53
Affect attunement, 30
Affection, 126
Affiliation, 190
Aggression, 57
Anarchy, 69, 102, 194
Anzieu, 18, 23, 26, 46, 159, 199
Appreciation, 166
Assimilation, 202–215
Attachment, 157
Autonomous group, 54
Awareness, 22

Bach, 56, 57
Bales, 114, 143
Basic assumption group, 1, 13, 30
Bateson, 53, 77
Belonging, 113–114, 127, 156, 182, 212–213
Benne and Sheats, 22
Bennis and Shepard, 16, 56
Berkowitz and Walster, 181
Berne, 101

Bettelheim, 54
Between, The, 182, 185
Bion, 1, 3, 7, 14, 22, 30, 56, 65, 98, 125, 118
Blake, 128
Blake and Mouton, 179
Bowlby, 156–157
Bradford, 9, 15, 33
Brown, 146
Buber, 51, 82, 109
Burns and Stalker, 68
Buss and Portnoy, 182
Byrne, 180

Campbell, 37
Cannibalism, 184
Cartwright and Zander, 179, 203
Casement, 193
Categories of intervention, 110
Categorization of personality, 143
Causality, 139, 174–175
Chastity, 139, 174–175
Cocoon of goodness, 199
Co-creation, 204
Cohesion, 42
Cohn, 111, 126
Collaboration, 153
Collective unconscious, 97

Community, 35
Community meeting, 146
Confirming, 110
Conflict, 148
Confluence, 168, 182
Confluent Dialogue, 113, 115
Contact boundary, 33, 44, 173, 204
Contact Dialogue, 113
Contact phase, 113
Contact skills between groups, 199
Contesting, 110
Continuity, 149
Control, 59
Cornering power, 153
Creative adjustment, 64
Creative competition, 203–204
Cycle of Experience, 136, 204

De Mare, 110, 126, 211
Deep-level processing, 114
Definition of the ingroup, 176
Deliberation, 64
Dependent pairing, 125
Despotism, 70
Destruction, 131
De-structuring, 58, 131, 141
Determinism, 36, 207–208
Developmental theory, 88, 142–143
Dialogue, 3, 101, 104, 107–113, 114–115, 120, 148
Differentiation, 59
Disintegration, 141
Displacement activity, 120
Double bind, 68
Dreams, 214
Dreams and the group, 55
Dream-telling, 60–63, 102, 103–104
Dynamical whole, 179, 180

Eating, 43
Economy of time, 141–142
Efran, Lukens and Lukens, 8
Egalitarian myth, 9
Ego-processes, 57
Eliot, 135, 148
Emergent Self, 30
Empty ground, 74
Enchantment, 54
Endless groups, 210
Entropy, 131
Environment, 163
Environment Dialogue, 113
Ephemeral groups, 210
Equifinality, 69
Equity, Theory, 181
Erickson, 43
Erikson, 149
Exclusion, 43
Experiential learning, 159

Fear, 212, 213
Feder, 98
Feder and Ronall, 2
Festinger, 179, 180
Field, 77–81
Fight and flight, 13, 56
Final contact, 159, 170, 171, 185
Fixed-gestalt, 93
Follow-up to groups, 198
Fore-contact, 16
Foulkes, 21, 47, 97, 156
Foulkes and Anthony, 3
Fragmentation terror, 65
Free dialogue, 112
Freud, 19, 56, 142, 143, 157, 161, 204
Frew, 18, 56, 110
Friedman, 109, 182
Fusion, 168

Gleick, 177
Goffman, 18

Index

Goldstein, 3, 43, 73, 199
Good faith, 51
Goodman, 3, 127, 171
Group agreement, 95
Group and individual, 205
Group-as-a-whole, 97
Group as entity, 87, 94, 99
Group boundary, 173
Group-centred consciousness, 189
Group consciousness, 150
Group contact boundary, 209
Group death, 144
Group fragmentation, 199
Group identity, 19
Group Illusion, The, 159, 171
Group membership, 127
Group-mind, 97
Group mood, 6
Group skin, 174, 185
Group therapy, 64
Group trance, 52, 55
Gustafson and Cooper, 11, 144, 148

Handy, 59
Harrison, 71
Healthy confluence, 109, 170
Herschel, 202
Heterogeneity, 85, 129, 190, 215
Hic et nunc, 21
Hierarchical tendency, 73
Hierarchy of gestalt formation, 128, 212
Hierarchy of needs, 443
Homosexual sub-group, 56
Hostility, 8, 155
Houston, 2, 208
Hypnosis, 161

I-Thou, 109, 110, 137
Id and ego, 214

Id-process, 57
Illusion of goodness, 49
Immortality, 141
Imposition, 60, 110
Impulse, 64
Inclusion, 18
Individuation, 177
Indivisibility, 186
In-group, 33
Initial conditions, 1, 3, 177
In-love state, 173, 182
Integration of group theories, 210–211
Interactive gestalt, 3
Interactive interdependence, 181
Interdependence, 182
Inter-group, 147
Intergroup contact boundary, 157
Inter-group event, 92
Inter-group meeting, 42
Inter-group rivalry, 153, 156, 174, 176
Interpretation and gestalt, 23
Interpretations, 53
Intersubjectivity, 30, 163
Intimacy system, 15, 71
Intrapsychic dialogue, 111, 112
Introjection, 43, 74

James, 64
Jung, 35, 111, 117

Kelly, 19
Klein, 6, 35, 52
Knopf, 152, 182–183
Kohut, 78, 142
Koinonia, 211
Kreeger, 166

Lacunae, 38
Large gestalt, 16

Large groups, 147–148
Last Supper, The, 51
Law of Praegnanz, 15, 85, 129, 157
Leadership, 59, 60
Leary, 190
Le Bon, 157
Levinson, 210
Lewin, 3, 77, 99, 179, 202
Lifton, 171
Loss of individuality, 157, 168, 174
Love and AMORA, 211–212, 213
Love as cohesive force, 161
Lynch-mob, 95

Machiavelli, 164
Martin and Saljo, 114
Marx, 47
Maslow, 19
McDougall, 157, 175
Mechanistic groups, 68
Median group, 7
Meetings between groups, 187
Merleau-Ponty, 121
Merry and Brown, 77
Messianic promise, 65
Microsphere, 34
Miller and Rice, 77
Milner, 34
Minuchin, 11
Mitchell, 140, 197
Monarchy, 155
Mood of expectation, 125
Morris, 35
Mother-group, 38, 43
Mourning, 141
Multiple membership, 83, 122, 127
Multiple pairings

Nevis, 136, 140, 154, 204
Nevis and Zinker, 71

New configurations, 144
Nichols, 11
Nodal points, 159, 166
Now as microcosm, 209

O, 26, 29, 31, 37, 38
Object relations, 163
Oceanic consciousness, 63
O'Leary, 203
Open Systems, 102
Orne, 42
Outcome, 151
Out-group, 33, 44, 77, 144, 147, 185
Outsiders, 161

Pairing, 65, 117, 180–181
Palmer, 162
Palo Alto School, 67
Paralinguistics, 34
Pathogenic logic, 67, 68
Pearce and Cronen, 68
Pecking order, 18
Perls, 2, 16, 19, 22, 23, 43, 51, 53, 58, 66, 131, 184
Perls, Hefferline and Goodman, 84, 128, 191, 193, 195, 197
Personality, 195
Petty victory, 51
Phallic mother, 54
Phases of group life, 56
Phenomena and now, 35
Phenomenology, 1, 105, 120, 152, 108
Philomenon, 164
Plato, 48, 66, 107
Plato's army, 151
Polarity, 57, 106
Political therapy, 99
Politics and group structure, 71–72

Index

Politics and therapy, 99
Polster, 98, 148
Positive re-framing, 11
Post-contact, 141, 185–186, 189, 200
Power of the secretariat, 47
Power system, 15, 71
Pre-verbal glimpse, 79
Primal horde, 19
Projective identification, 207

Recapitulation of development, 143
Reference group, 83
Response-ability, 80, 83
Responsibility, 127
Retroflection, 94
Rice, 68
Rogers, 6, 161
Rossi, 52

Samuels, 179
Sartre, 51, 133
Satir, 6
Schumacher, 183
Schutz, 7, 18, 125
Selective authenticity, 126
Self, 19, 197
Self-categorisation, 174
Self-conquest, 66, 94
Self-regulation, 159
Selvini-Palozzoli, 68
Sense of belonging, 190
Separate to integrate, 56, 57
Sexualised contact, 179
Sexualised feeling, 127
Significant missing elements, 30
Simkin, 114
Simmel, 117, 180
Skynner and Cleese, 143
Small group, 16

Snow, 164
Sociogram, 178
Solidarity, 156
Sovereign groups, 153
Spontaneity, 64
Stern, 15, 30, 82, 84, 143, 163
Sub-grouping, 46
Sullivan, 19, 104
Superego of group, 181
Survival, 18
Synchronicity, 117

Thaeatetus, 48, 107
Theme or meta-topic, 60
Therapeutic dialogue, 112
Therapeutic distance, 64
Therapy as service, 98–99
Thibaut and Kelley, 191
Thompson, 78
Thurber's War, 46, 56
Tradition, 152, 156
Transactional analysis, 179
Transference, 96, 124, 136, 193, 207
Transference to group, 206–207
Treatment of network, 166
Tribal responses, 156
True pairing, 125
Turner, 174
Turquet, 85, 125, 148, 168

Unconscious group dynamics, 98
Underdog, 152
Unfinished gestalts, 198
Unifying vocabulary, 164
Unpossessive love, 150
Us and Them, 144

Verbal self, 82
von Bertalanffy, 116

War, 33
War between the sexes, 52
War-strategy, 151
Waves and particles, 136–137
Weir, 38
Wheeler, 113
White, 10
Whole-group, 57
Wholeness, 204
Wide gestalt, 70, 156, 189
Wilder, 177

Winnicott, 143
Withdrawing, 169
Worchel, 177
Work group, 13, 55

Yalom, 43
Yontef, 74

Zinker, 98, 160